D0810932

Atlas of
Bedside
Procedures

Atlas of Bedside Procedures

Thomas J. Vander Salm, M.D., Editor
Associate Professor of Surgery,
University of Massachusetts Medical School, Worcester

Bruce S. Cutler, M.D., Coeditor
Associate Professor of Surgery,
University of Massachusetts Medical School, Worcester

H. Brownell Wheeler, M.D., Coeditor
Professor and Chairman, Department of Surgery,
University of Massachusetts Medical School, Worcester

Medical Illustrators
Charles H. Boyter, M.S.M.I.
Marcia Williams, M.S.M.I.
Douglas Patrick Russell

Foreword by **W. Gerald Austen, M.D.**
Edward D. Churchill Professor of Surgery,
Harvard Medical School; Chief of Surgery,
Massachusetts General Hospital, Boston

Little, Brown and Company   Boston

Copyright © 1979 by Little, Brown and Company (Inc.)

First Edition

Fifth Printing

All rights reserved. No part of this book may be reproduced in any form or by any electronic or mechanical means, including information storage and retrieval systems, without permission in writing from the publisher, except by a reviewer who may quote brief passages in a review.

Library of Congress Catalog Card No. 79-65313

ISBN 0-316-89605-5

Printed in the United States of America

HAL

109959

BELMONT COLLEGE LIBRARY

To Jessica and Jamie

Contents

Foreword

During the last three decades, in-hospital medicine has become progressively more effective yet at the same time, quite naturally, more complicated. The day of medicine by intuition has gradually changed to medicine based on documentation and physiological understanding. While many procedures require an operating room situation, there has gradually grown up a large number of important diagnostic and therapeutic procedures that can and should be done at the bedside. Some of these procedures are quite simple and others are more complicated, but when done properly, they all make a tremendous difference in the care of the patient.

This atlas of bedside procedures has been developed to aid the physician in the management of the patient for whom these bedside procedures are appropriate. The authors have chosen 40 procedures that appear to be most necessary and important, and have developed a specific approach for each procedure with indications, extensive schematic representations of specific technique, and complications and their treatment. They have presented a particular technique in each case, preferring to indicate their method of choice rather than to present multiple methods. Similarly, they have compiled a modest bibliography pertinent to each situation that they discuss, and have not tried to present an exhaustive bibliography.

Each of the techniques presented is important and, used in the right situation and in the right way, will be of great assistance in proper management of the patient. Each procedure can be well done at the bedside, and if handled in the manner described in the atlas, the procedure should go well and be quite helpful in the care of the patient.

W. Gerald Austen

Preface

There is a childhood game called Telephone in which a "secret" is passed by word of mouth from one child to another. The last in line repeats the secret out loud to the entire group. The distortion that occurs is usually so striking that everyone laughs.

Like the childhood game of Telephone, important details about patient procedures are often passed along orally from one physician to another, with inevitable distortion in the information transmitted. The unfortunate consequence is that unnecessary and sometimes serious complications occur following so-called minor procedures.

In 1975 we were planning to open a new surgical service in the recently completed University of Massachusetts Hospital. We were anxious that each patient care procedure be performed as well as possible. We had learned (sometimes from painful experience) that patients can encounter serious problems from complications due to unsupervised or poorly taught bedside procedures carried out by inexperienced physicians or residents. We decided to put an explicit, up-to-date, and authoritative atlas of bedside procedures on every clinical ward, in the emergency room, and in the outpatient areas of our new hospital. To our surprise we could not find such an atlas; we therefore decided to write the book ourselves.

This atlas describes a standard technique for 40 of the most common and important bedside procedures. To present the information in the clearest and most succinct fashion, we have relied on an outline format with many line drawings. The indications and contraindications for each procedure are specified. The major complications are enumerated, together with their causes and the best means of avoiding those causes. The bibliography is short, pertinent, and annotated—the format we believe most useful to our readers. An appendix lists the equipment needed for each procedure in the most logical order of preparation. Nursing personnel will find this appendix helpful when gathering equipment for these procedures or when establishing permanent sets for the procedures most frequently performed. An equipment list accompanies each chapter. It contains the same items as the appendix but listed in the order of use, thus facilitating organization of the procedure.

Any procedure may be performed in various ways. We make no claim that the techniques described herein are the only proper ones—simply that they have worked well for us, that they minimize complications, and that they ensure a high degree of success. We believe that the ready availability of an authoritative and clearly illustrated method will help residents and medical students learn to perform these procedures. This atlas should also prove useful to emergency room physicians or any other medical personnel called upon to carry out or assist in procedures with which they are unfamiliar.

We are indebted to many individuals for their contributions to this atlas. We are particularly proud of the superbly clear drawings. Any success achieved by this work must be largely attributed to our artists and illustrators—Charles H. Boyter, Marcia Williams, Douglas Patrick Russell, and their associates. We are most appreciative of their patience with our many last-minute changes. Lin Richter, the medical editor-in-chief at Little, Brown and Company, and her staff worked with us from the inception of this book through every arduous step along the way to completion. Not only did her enthusiasm keep the work going when our spirits flagged but all our meetings with her were unfailingly pleasant and productive. Wendy Perry and Sharon Margolin typed, retyped, and yet again uncomplainingly retyped a manuscript that was often altered. We are deeply indebted to them and also to Beverly Greene, who performed our editing, indexing, and proofreading expertly and efficiently. We also thank Paul Cardullo who patiently posed for most of our drawings.

Finally, we owe a particular debt of gratitude to those individuals who taught us the material presented herein. They include our own former teachers and professional associates. We would especially like to acknowledge our indebtedness to Dr. W. Gerald Austen, not only for past training but also for his kindness in providing a foreword to this book. Specialty consultants have provided the necessary experience for procedures with which we were personally unfamiliar, and have been invaluable in their contributions. Last and most particularly, we acknowledge our humble indebtedness to many former patients who have taught us through their clinical course when and how these procedures should be done.

T. J. V.
B. S. C.
H. B. W.

Contributors

Carlton M. Akins, M.D.
Associate Professor of Orthopedic Surgery,
University of Massachusetts Medical School, Worcester

Bruce S. Cutler, M.D.
Associate Professor of Surgery,
University of Massachusetts Medical School, Worcester

Robin I. Davidson, M.D.
Associate Professor of Neurosurgery,
Section of Neurosurgery, Department of Surgery,
University of Massachusetts Medical School, Worcester

Gregory L. Eastwood, M.D.
Associate Professor of Medicine,
University of Massachusetts Medical School, Worcester

Garry F. Fitzpatrick, M.D.
Assistant Professor of Surgery,
University of Massachusetts Medical School, Worcester

Richard R. Gacek, M.D.
Professor and Chairman, Department of Otolaryngology,
State University of New York, Upstate Medical Center,
College of Medicine, Syracuse

Thomas F. Halpin, M.D.
Assistant Professor of Obstetrics and Gynecology,
University of Massachusetts Medical School, Worcester

Timothy B. Hopkins, M.D.
Instructor in Surgery,
University of Massachusetts Medical School, Worcester

John P. Howe III, M.D.
Associate Professor of Medicine and Chief of Staff,
University of Massachusetts Medical School, Worcester

Ira S. Ockene, M.D.
Associate Professor of Medicine,
University of Massachusetts Medical School, Worcester

John A. Paraskos, M.D.
Associate Professor of Medicine,
University of Massachusetts Medical School, Worcester

Liberto Pechet, M.D.
Professor of Medicine and of Pathology, Department of Medicine,
University of Massachusetts Medical School, Worcester

Peter G. Pletka, M.D.
Associate Professor of Medicine,
University of Massachusetts Medical School, Worcester

Joel M. Seidman, M.D.
Associate Professor of Medicine and of Physiology,
University of Massachusetts Medical School, Worcester

Adrian S. Selwyn, M.D.
Attending Anaesthesiologist, Department of Anaesthesia,
Royal Prince Alfred Hospital, Camperdown, Australia;
formerly Associate Professor of Anaesthesia,
University of Massachusetts Medical School, Worcester

Wayne E. Silva, M.D.
Associate Professor of Surgery,
University of Massachusetts Medical School, Worcester

Thomas J. Vander Salm, M.D.
Associate Professor of Surgery,
University of Massachusetts Medical School, Worcester

H. Brownell Wheeler, M.D.
Professor and Chairman, Department of Surgery,
University of Massachusetts Medical School, Worcester

Atlas of
Bedside
Procedures

Notice

The indications and dosages of all drugs in this book have been recommended in the medical literature and conform to the practices of the general medical community. The medications described do not necessarily have specific approval by the Food and Drug Administration for use in the diseases and dosages for which they are recommended. The package insert for each drug should be consulted for use and dosage as approved by the FDA. Because standards for usage change, it is advisable to keep abreast of revised recommendations, particularly those concerning new drugs.

1.
Peripheral Intravenous Cannulation

Method of Bruce S. Cutler

INDICATIONS

Intravenous administration of drugs and fluids

EQUIPMENT (see Appendix for sample kit)

Skin prep

    Alcohol-acetone swab

    Povidone-iodine swab

Cannulation equipment

    Intravenous solution, tubing, and stand

    Needle, 14-gauge × 1½-inch

    Intravenous cannula

      Butterfly needle

      or

      Plastic cannula

        Over-the-needle cannula (Angiocath)

        or

        Through-the-needle cannula (Intracath)

    Tourniquet

Local anesthesia

    Plastic syringe, 3-ml

    Needle, 25-gauge × ⅝-inch

    Lidocaine 1%, 5 ml

Dressing

    Povidone-iodine ointment

    Sterile gauze

    Adhesive tape, 1-inch

    Armboard

PREPARATION TECHNIQUE

1. Select intravenous site

Apply venous tourniquet to upper arm.

Instruct patient to open and close fist to distend veins.

Select palpable vein on dorsum of hand or forearm; preserve more proximal veins for later use.

2. Prep skin

Cleanse skin over vein with alcohol-acetone swab.

Prep same area with povidone-iodine swab.

3. Anesthetize skin (for large-bore intravenous needles only)

Inject 1% lidocaine at intended puncture site.

Do not puncture vein.

4. Prepare ancillary equipment

Fill intravenous tubing with solution; replace sterile cap over connector.

Prepare several pieces of 1-inch adhesive tape to secure intravenous cannula.

TECHNIQUE OF INSERTION OF BUTTERFLY NEEDLE

1. Select and prepare butterfly needle of appropriate size

Remove tubular needle protector.

Loosen sterile cap from free end to permit blood to return through tubing.

Figure 1

2. Stabilize position of vein in subcutaneous tissue

Apply traction to skin with thumb of nondominant hand.

Hold two wings of scalp vein needle together with bevel of needle upward.

Figure 1

3. Puncture skin

Hold needle at 15-degree angle to skin.

Figure 2

4. Puncture vein

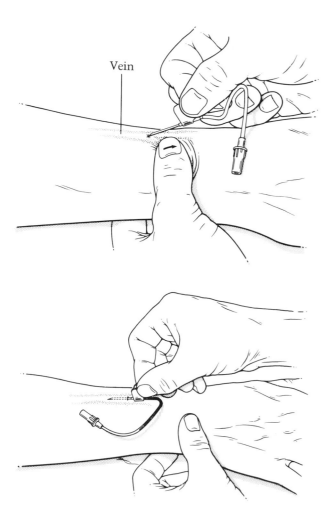

Vein

Figure 1
Stabilize vein in subcutaneous tissue; puncture skin.

Figure 2
Puncture vein.

Identify entry by return of blood in tubing.

Advance needle full length.

Keep needle tip in vein lumen.

If hematoma develops, stop, withdraw needle, loosen tourniquet, apply local pressure, and select new site.

5. Release tourniquet

6. Start infusion

7. Apply dressing

Apply povidone-iodine ointment to puncture site.

Apply sterile gauze dressing.

Figure 3

Secure with adhesive tape.

Use armboard to immobilize wrist or elbow if necessary.

TECHNIQUE OF INSERTION OF OVER-THE-NEEDLE CANNULA (Angiocath)

1. Select cannula size appropriate for available vein and for type and rate of solution to be infused

Remember that blood will not flow easily through cannula smaller than 18-gauge.

Ascertain that cannula slides easily over needle-obturator.

Loosen plug in needle hub to permit backflow of blood.

2. Anesthetize skin

Inject lidocaine 1% at intended puncture site.

Avoid puncture of vein.

Figure 4

3. Stabilize vein in subcutaneous tissue

Apply traction to skin with thumb of nondominant hand.

Figure 4

4. Puncture skin

For large-bore cannulas, prepuncture skin with 14-gauge needle to avoid cannula binding on skin.

Slide skin to one side of vein to avoid puncturing vein.

Insert Angiocath at 15-degree angle with skin.

Figure 5

5. Puncture vein

Advance needle and cannula as a unit until vein is punctured.

Identify vein entry by free backflow of blood.

Advance needle *and cannula* 5 mm into vein.

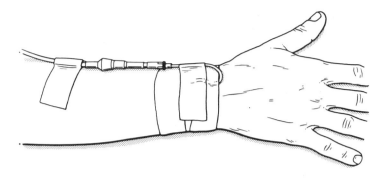

Figure 3
Apply dressing.

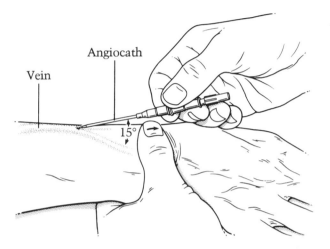

Vein

Angiocath

15°

Figure 4
Stabilize vein in subcutaneous tissue; puncture skin.

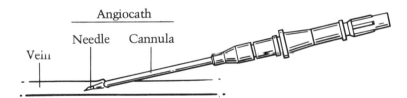

Angiocath

Needle   Cannula

Vein

Figure 5
Puncture vein.

Figure 6

6. Advance cannula into vein

Hold hub of needle with thumb and forefinger and slide catheter over needle into vein.

Remove needle.

Free backflow of blood indicates satisfactory intravenous position.

Apply pressure over vein at cannula tip to control bleeding.

If catheter fails to enter vein, do not attempt to reinsert needle into cannula; remove entire device and start again.

7. Release tourniquet

8. Attach intravenous tubing to hub of cannula

9. Start infusion

Free flow of fluid indicates satisfactory cannulation.

If swelling or hematoma develops, stop, remove cannula, apply local pressure, and select a new site.

10. Apply dressing

Apply povidone-iodine ointment to puncture site.

Apply sterile gauze dressing.

Secure with adhesive tape.

Use armboard to immobilize wrist or elbow if necessary.

TECHNIQUE OF INSERTION OF THROUGH-THE-NEEDLE CANNULA (Intracath)

1. Anesthetize skin

Anesthetize at intended puncture site.

Avoid puncture of vein.

2. Select cannula size appropriate for available vein and type and rate of solution to be infused

Remember that blood will not flow easily through cannula smaller than 16-gauge (Large Intracath).

Remove tubular needle protector.

Ascertain that inner cannula does not project from needle.

Figure 7

3. Stabilize position of vein in subcutaneous tissue

Apply traction to skin with thumb of nondominant hand.

Figure 7

4. Puncture skin

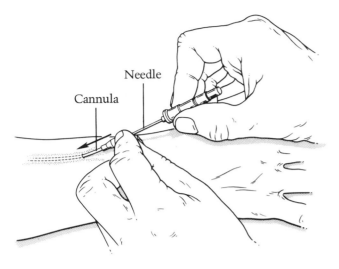

Cannula

Needle

Figure 6
Advance cannula into vein.

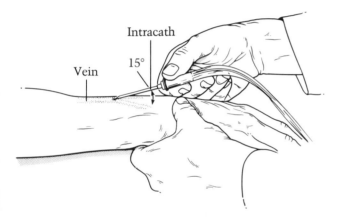

Vein

Intracath

15°

Figure 7
Stabilize vein in subcutaneous tissue; puncture skin.

Figure 8

5. Puncture vein

Advance needle containing cannula until vein is entered.

Advance needle 5 mm into vein.

Return of blood through cannula confirms intravenous location.

Figure 9

6. Advance cannula into vein

Hold junction of needle hub and plastic cannula sheath with thumb and forefinger, and slide cannula through needle into vein.

Engage hub of cannula into hub of needle.

7. Release tourniquet

Figure 10

8. Prepare cannula for infusion

Withdraw cannula 2 cm, remove plastic cannula sheath and stylette, and apply needle protector.

9. Attach intravenous tubing to hub of cannula

10. Start infusion

Free flow of fluid indicates satisfactory cannulation.

If swelling or hematoma develops, stop, remove cannula, apply local pressure, and select new site.

11. Apply dressing

Apply povidone-iodine ointment to puncture site.

Apply sterile gauze dressing.

Secure with adhesive tape.

Use armboard to immobilize wrist or elbow if necessary.

COMPLICATIONS

Hematoma

Etiology

Through-and-through puncture of vein or laceration of vein wall.

Prevention

Use oblique angle when advancing needle into vein.

After failed attempt, release tourniquet, try new location.

Phlebitis

Etiology

Infusion of hypertonic or irritating drugs.

Prevention

Use isotonic solutions; dilute concentrations of drugs known to cause phlebitis, or use a central intravenous site.

Change IV sites frequently.

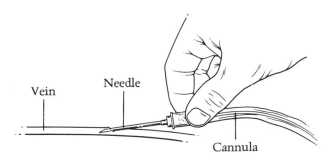

Vein   Needle

Cannula

Figure 8
Puncture vein.

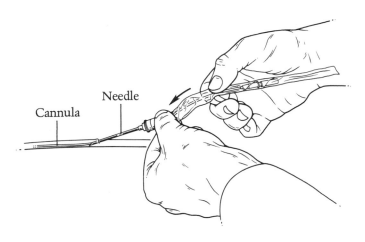

Cannula   Needle

Figure 9
Advance cannula into
vein.

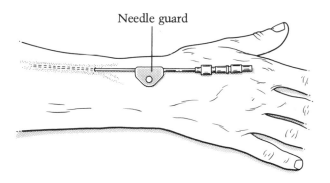

Needle guard

Figure 10
Prepare cannula for
infusion.

Catheter embolism

Etiology

Shear-off of Intracath cannula during an attempt to slide cannula back through needle.

Prevention

Remove cannula and needle as single unit following failed venipuncture prior to second try; do not slide cannula back through Intracath needle.

Infiltration

Etiology

Needle or cannula not in vein.

Prevention

Avoid placing intravenous devices over joints.

Use armboard to stabilize joints.

Restrain uncooperative patients.

Remove cannula at first sign of infiltration.

Sepsis

Etiology

Break in sterile technique during placement.

Contamination of puncture wound after placement due to improper dressing technique.

Prevention

Properly cleanse and prep skin.

Maintain sterile technique while placing intravenous cannula.

Apply povidone-iodine ointment to puncture site.

CARE OF INTRAVENOUS LINES

Check frequently for infiltration, phlebitis, or sepsis.

Change dressings used with plastic cannulas, and reapply povidone-iodine ointment daily.

SELECTED BIBLIOGRAPHY

1. Duma, R. J., Warner, J. F., and Dalton, H. P. Septicemia from intravenous infusions. *N. Engl. J. Med.* 284:257, 1971.

   Discussions of the septic hazards of intravenous therapy.

2. Keeley, J. L. Intravenous injections and infusions. *Am. J. Surg.* 50:485, 1940.

   An older, but excellent, description of intravenous technique and venous cutdown.

3. Macht, D. I. The history of intravenous and subcutaneous administration of drugs. *J.A.M.A.* 66:856, 1916.

   An historical review of intravenous techniques.

2.
Venous Cutdown

Method of
Thomas J. Vander Salm

INDICATIONS

Vein cannulation when percutaneous method not feasible

EQUIPMENT (see Appendix for sample kit)

Skin prep

Sterile sponges

Alcohol-acetone solution

Povidone-iodine solution

Sterile field

Mask, gown, gloves

Towels, towel clips

Local anesthetic

Syringe, 2-ml

Needles

25-gauge × ⅝-inch

22-gauge × 1½-inch

Lidocaine 1%, 10 ml

Cutdown equipment

Sterile sponges

Syringes, 10-ml

Knife handle, #3

Scalpel blades, #11, #15

Retractor

    Small self-retaining

    Small rake, 2

Forceps

    Fine-toothed

    Smooth

Scissors

    Suture

    Metzenbaum

    Curved iris

Clamps

    Curved and straight mosquito, 5

Needle holder

Cutdown catheter assortment, Silastic preferred

Needle, 14-gauge × 1½-inch

Ligatures, 3-0 silk

Sutures, skin

Injectable saline, 30-ml vial

Dressing

    Povidone-iodine ointment

    Sponges

    Tincture of benzoin

    Adhesive tape

Infusion

    Intravenous solution, tubing, and stand

Figure 1

POSITION

Supine, for one of the following veins:

    Saphenous vein at ankle

    Saphenous vein at groin

    Antecubital veins, basilic or cephalic

    Cephalic vein in deltopectoral groove

    External jugular vein

    Internal jugular vein (see Chapter 5)

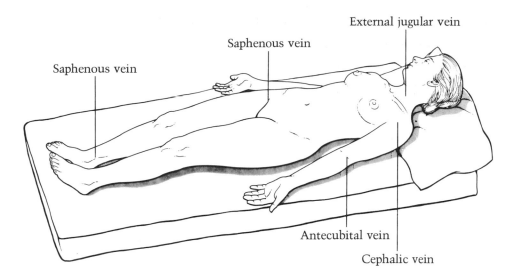

Saphenous vein

Saphenous vein

External jugular vein

Antecubital vein

Cephalic vein

Figure 1
Position: common cut-
down sites.

TECHNIQUE (only saphenous vein cutdown at ankle shown; others similar)

Figure 2

    1. Use mask, gown, and gloves

    2. Prep and drape appropriate area

    3. Infiltrate local anesthetic

Figure 3

    4. Incise skin and subcutaneous tissue

    Make transverse incision over vein.

    For saphenous vein at ankle, 1.5 cm anterior and cephalad to medial malleolus.

Figure 4

    5. Isolate vein

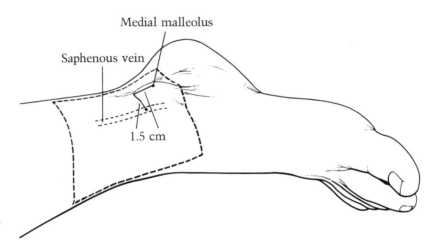

Figure 2
Prep and drape appropriate area.

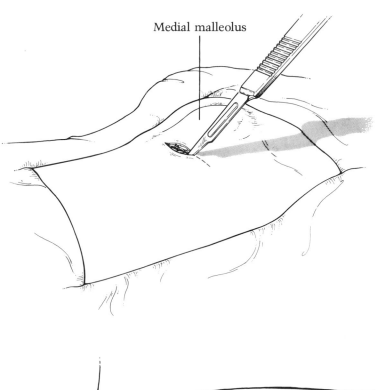

Medial malleolus

Figure 3
Incise skin and subcutaneous tissue.

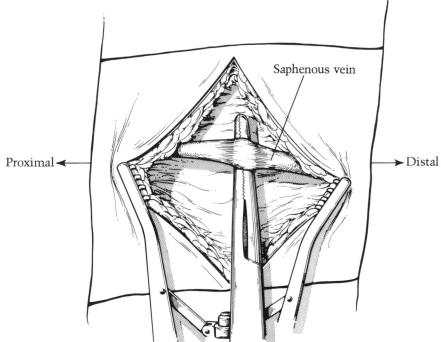

Saphenous vein

Proximal ◄———————————————► Distal

Figure 4
Isolate vein.

Figure 5

6. Pass two ligatures beneath vein

Tie distal ligature.

Figure 6

7. Select cannula of appropriate size

For ease of insertion, bevel tip and round off point.

8. Bring cannula through separate stab wound (omit in emergency situations)

Figure 7A

Pass 14-gauge needle through skin, from inside out.

Pass cannula through needle, from outside in.

Figure 7B

Remove needle.

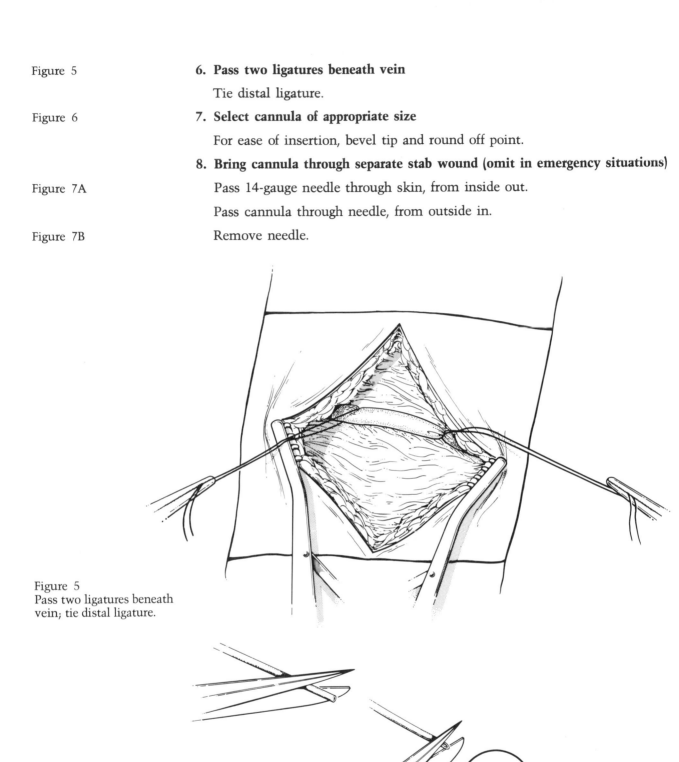

Figure 5
Pass two ligatures beneath
vein; tie distal ligature.

Figure 6
Select and bevel appro-
priate size cannula.

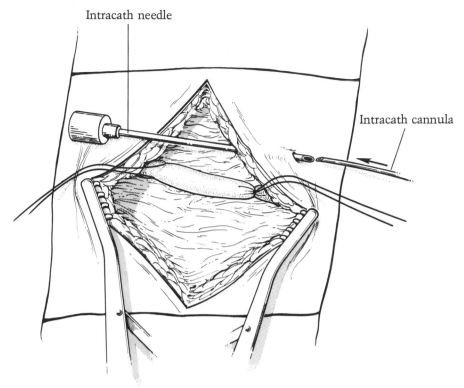

Intracath needle

Intracath cannula

A

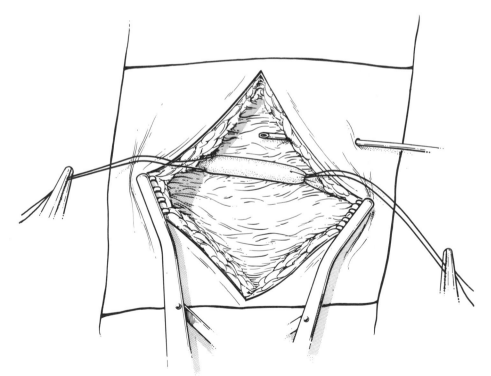

B

Figure 7
Bring cannula through
separate stab wound.

17

Figure 8

9. Perform venotomy

Incise vein halfway through with #11 blade.

Angle incision distally and superficially.

Figure 9

Alternatively, cannulate vein with needle through which (Intracath) or over which (Angiocath) a plastic cannula may be threaded. This obviates incising vein.

Figure 10

10. Insert cannula

Bevel facing back wall.

Relax proximal ligature.

Gently advance cannula.

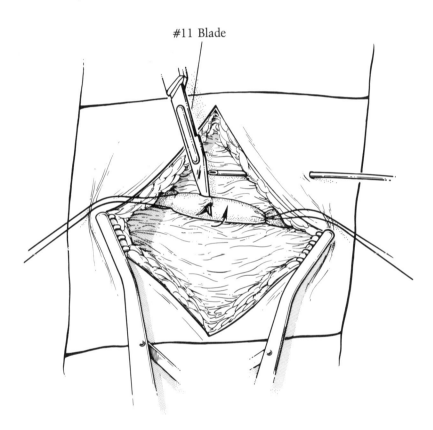

#11 Blade

Figure 8
Perform venotomy.

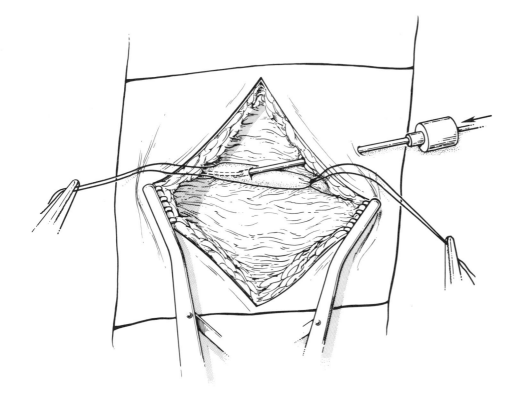

Figure 9
Perform venotomy, alternate method.

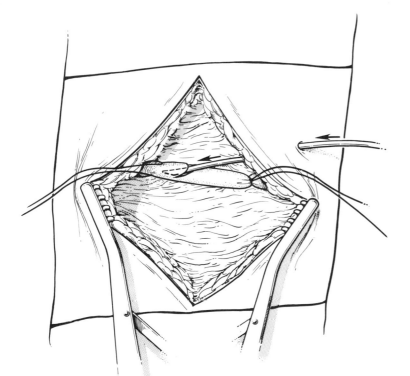

Figure 10
Insert cannula.

Figure 11

11. Aspirate, then flush cannula

Use saline-filled syringe.

Aspirate to confirm free flow of blood.

Flush to prevent blood clotting in cannula.

Figure 11

12. Secure cannula in vein

Tie proximal ligature.

Reaspirate and flush cannula to confirm patency.

Figure 12

13. Close wound

Suture cannula to skin at exit point.

Suture skin.

Reconfirm cannula patency.

Figure 13

14. Apply dressing

Apply povidone-iodine ointment to wound.

Apply sterile gauze dressing.

Tape cannula and occlusive dressing securely.

15. Begin infusion

Remove syringe, attach intravenous tubing.

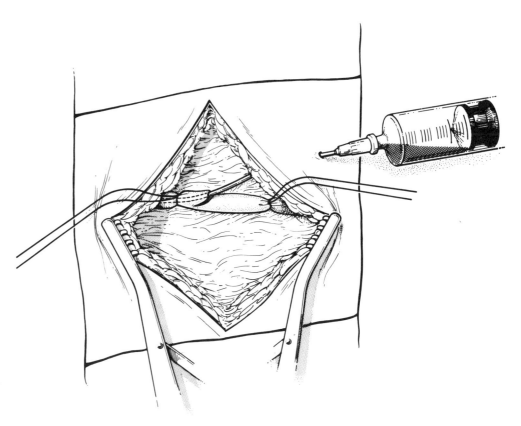

Figure 11
Aspirate, then flush cannula. Secure cannula in vein.

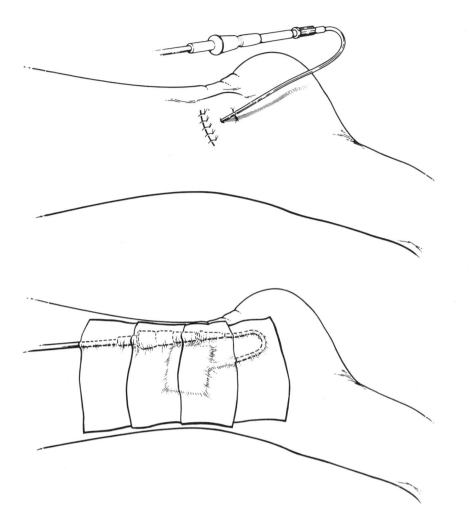

Figure 12
Close wound, suture
cannula.

Figure 13
Apply dressing.

COMPLICATIONS

Infection

Etiology

Wound contamination.

Prevention

Use strict asepsis.

Bring cannula out through stab wound.

Avoid long dwell time.

Care for catheter as under Subclavian Vein Cannulation (Chapter 3).

Thrombophlebitis

Etiology

Sepsis (wound contamination).

Mechanical or chemical irritation of vein wall.

Prevention

See under Infection.

Use Silastic cannula instead of polyethylene cannula.

Dilute solutions known to cause phlebitis.

Arterial cannulation

Etiology

Mistaking artery for vein.

Prevention

A problem only in infants, in whom arteries and veins are difficult to differentiate grossly, or in patients in shock.

Ascertain absence of arterial pulsation.

Failure to find vein

Etiology

Previous thrombophlebitis, mistaking vein for tendons or nerve (especially a thick walled saphenous vein), venous spasm, previous vein stripping.

Prevention

Do not attempt cutdown after previous thrombophlebitis or vein stripping.

Use gentle technique to avoid spasm.

SELECTED BIBLIOGRAPHY

1. Bogen, J.   Local complications in 167 patients with indwelling venous catheters. *Surg. Gynecol. Obstet.* 110:112, 1960.

   Documents the increasing number of complications (primarily thrombophlebitis) with increasing dwell time of the cannula.

2. Keeley, J. L.   Intravenous injection and infusion. *Am. J. Surg.* 50:485, 1940.

   Good description of the technique of cutdown, which used at that time a metal cannula.

3. Kirkham, J. H.   Infusion into the internal saphenous vein at the ankle. *Lancet* 2:815, 1945.

   An early paper on polyethylene cannulation of veins, written when the author was a house officer. It is still an excellent "how-to-do-it" source and includes the method for controlling the vein.

4. Moran, J. M., Atwood, R. P., and Rowe, M. I.   A clinical and bacteriologic study of infections associated with venous cutdowns. *N. Engl. J. Med.* 272:554, 1965.

   Study confirming the decreased incidence of local sepsis with daily application of antibiotic ointment to the wound.

5. Shiu, M. H.   A method for conservation of veins in the surgical cutdown. *Surg. Gynecol. Obstet.* 134:315, 1972.

   Good drawings of the method of vein cannulation through a needle without incising the vein.

3.
Subclavian Vein Cannulation

Method of
Thomas J. Vander Salm

INDICATIONS

Central venous pressure measurement

Hyperalimentation

Vasopressor administration

Establishment of emergency intravenous route

EQUIPMENT (see Appendix for sample kit)

Skin prep

Sterile sponges

Alcohol-acetone solution

Povidone-iodine solution

Sterile field

Mask, gown, gloves

Towels

Half sheet

Towel clips

Local anesthetic

3-ml plastic syringe with 22-gauge needle

Lidocaine 1%, 5 ml

Cannulation equipment

    3-ml (non-Luer-Lok) plastic syringe

    14-gauge Subclavian Jugular Catheter Set (Deseret)

    or

    14-gauge Intracath (Deseret), 12-inch

    Injectable saline

    Scissors, suture

    3-0 silk suture on Keith needle

Dressing

    Povidone-iodine ointment

    Sponges

    Tincture of benzoin

    Adhesive tape

        1-inch

        3-inch

Infusion

    Intravenous solution, tubing, and stand

Figure 1

POSITION

Supine

10–20 degrees Trendelenburg

Head turned to opposite side

Roll under shoulders

TECHNIQUE

Figure 1

Figure 2

1. Prep and drape neck

    Identify anatomical landmarks.

2. Use mask, gown, and gloves

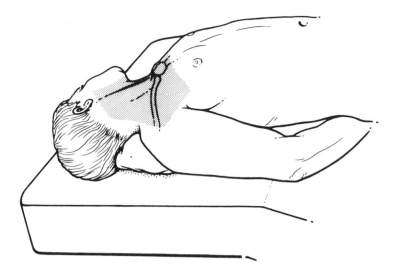

Figure 1
Position, prep, and drape
neck.

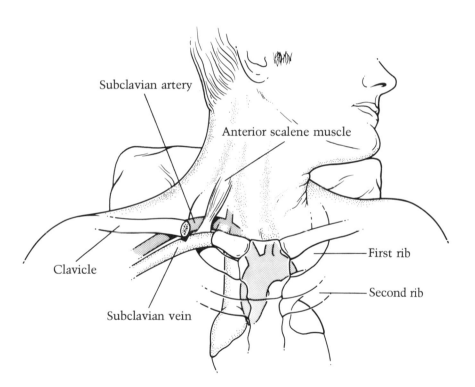

Subclavian artery

Anterior scalene muscle

First rib

Clavicle

Second rib

Subclavian vein

Figure 2
Identify anatomical land-
marks.

Figure 3

Figure 4

Figure 5

3. Infiltrate local anesthetic

Insert needle slightly lateral to midpoint of, and 2–3 cm caudal to, clavicle, to allow needle to pass under clavicle.

4. Insert cannulation (Intracath) needle (on non-Luer-Lok syringe) into same puncture site; aim for suprasternal notch

If patient on a ventilator, disconnect during this maneuver.

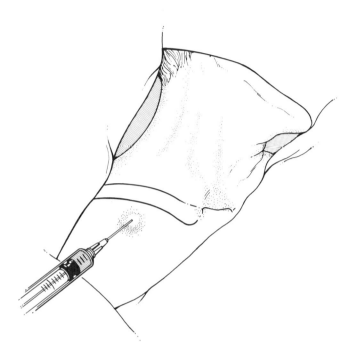

Figure 3
Infiltrate local anesthetic.

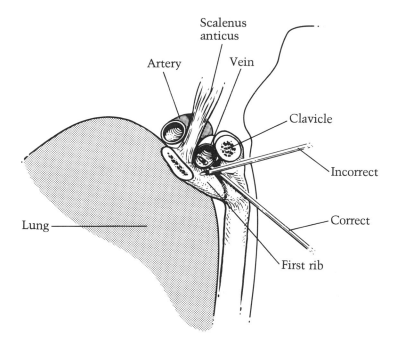

Artery

Scalenus anticus

Vein

Clavicle

Incorrect

Correct

Lung

First rib

Figure 4
Insert needle 2–3 cm
caudal to clavicle.

Suprasternal notch

Figure 5
Insert cannulation needle.
Aim for suprasternal
notch; aspirate.

Figure 5
Figure 6A
Figure 6B

5. Advance needle, aspirating gently; when venous blood returns freely, remove syringe and slide cannula through needle into subclavian vein

Confirm free return of venous blood during 360-degree axial rotation of needle.

Pulsatile resistance indicates subclavian artery—withdraw needle, repeat step 4.

Face needle bevel anterocaudally during cannula insertion.

Occlude needle hub with finger to prevent bleeding or air entrainment while preparing to insert cannula.

During cannula advancement, turn head back to ipsilateral side.

Maintain Trendelenburg position sufficiently steep to cause venous efflux from open needle.

Advance cannula into superior vena cava (about 15 cm in the adult).

Do not advance cannula if resistance encountered.

6. Withdraw needle, lock cannula and needle hubs together

With Subclavian Jugular Catheter, slide needle off cannula, screw hub onto cannula.

Apply needle guard if Intracath used.

Figure 7

7. Aspirate, then flush cannula with saline-filled syringe

Aspirate to confirm free flow of blood.

Flush to prevent blood clotting in cannula.

Figure 7

8. Suture cannula to skin

Repeat step 7 to confirm patency.

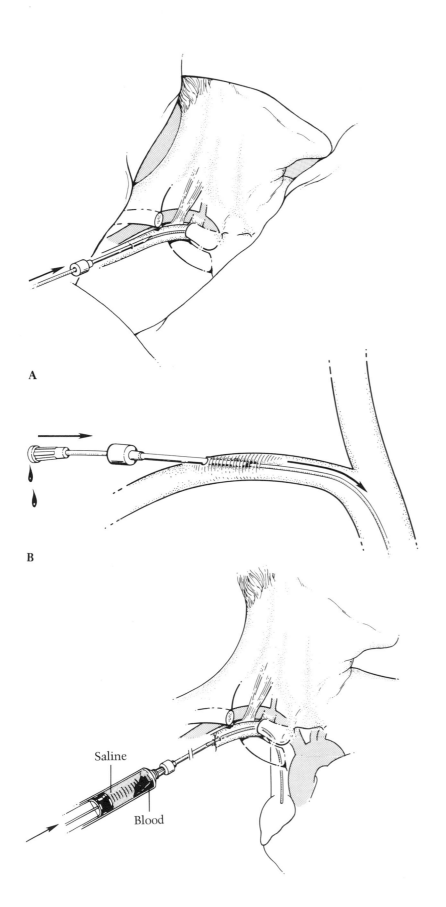

A

B

Figure 6
Advance needle, aspirating gently. When venous blood returns freely, remove syringe and slide cannula through needle into subclavian vein.

Saline

Blood

Figure 7
Aspirate, then flush cannula with saline filled syringe.

Figure 8

9. **Apply dressing**

Povidone-iodine ointment to puncture site.

Tincture of benzoin to surrounding skin.

Include needle and hub under dressing.

Tape securely.

10. **Begin infusion**

Remove syringe.

Attach cannula to intravenous tubing.

11. **Return bed to head-up position; assess for respiratory difficulty**

12. **Obtain chest x-ray**

Rule out hemothorax or pneumothorax.

Confirm cannula position in superior vena cava.

COMPLICATIONS

Pneumothorax

Etiology

Pleural laceration with air leak through needle.

Lung laceration.

Prevention

Abandon procedure after two unsuccessful attempts.

Avoid positive airway pressure during needle placement (remove patient from ventilator).

Keep syringe on needle until needle in vein.

Hemothorax

Etiology

Venous or arterial bleeding through pleural rent.

Prevention

Withdraw needle if pulsations felt through it.

Adhere to proper line of needle advancement (Technique, step 4).

Insert cannula gently to avoid pushing it through vein wall.

Abandon procedure after two unsuccessful attempts.

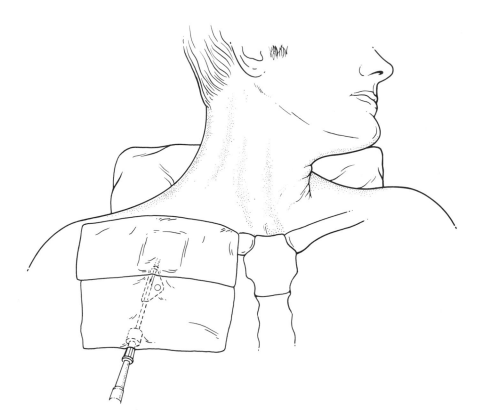

Figure 8
Apply dressing.

Hematoma

Etiology

Venous or arterial bleeding.

Prevention

Same as above.

Raise head of bed to reduce subclavian venous pressure at completion.

Hydrothorax or hydromediastinum

Etiology

Perforation of vein wall by cannula, thus administering perfusate into pleural space or mediastinum.

Prevention

Advance cannula gently; stop if resistance is encountered.

Air embolism

Etiology

Air entrained through open cannula or needle.

Prevention

Maintain sufficiently steep Trendelenburg position.

Open needle or cannula to atmosphere only briefly.

Cannula advancing up internal jugular vein

Etiology

Misdirected cannula; not always preventable.

Prevention

Face needle bevel anterocaudally during cannula advancement.

Turn head to ipsilateral side during cannula advancement, thereby increasing acuteness of subclavian–internal jugular vein angle.

Check cannula position with x-ray; replace if incorrect.

Subclavian vein thrombosis

Etiology

Catheter-induced phlebitis.

Prevention

Remove cannula as soon as possible.

Use less reactive Silastic cannula.

Catheter embolism

Etiology

    Cannula shearing off at needle tip.

    Cannula breaking off at skin.

Prevention

    Never withdraw cannula through needle.

    Prohibit cannula pivoting around skin entry site by secure taping.

Infection

Etiology

    Contamination either during insertion or dressing change or from blood-stream seeding.

Prevention

    Use meticulous asepsis in placing cannula and changing dressing.

    Remove cannula as soon as possible.

Myocardial puncture

Etiology

    Stiff polyethylene cannula impinging on endocardium.

Prevention

    Avoid excessive cannula advancement; confirm with x-ray.

    Substitute Silastic cannula for semirigid polyethylene cannula.

CARE OF SUBCLAVIAN LINE

Do not use "piggyback" IV lines

Daily: change IV tubing

Three times per week: change dressing

Remove dressing.

Use gloves and mask.

Prep with alcohol-acetone and povidone-iodine solution.

Apply povidone-iodine ointment to puncture site.

Apply new dressing.

Fever: if no source found, remove catheter

Culture blood peripherally and through catheter.

Culture catheter tip.

SELECTED BIBLIOGRAPHY

1. Aubaniac, R. L'injection intraveineuse sous-claviculaire. Avantages et techniques. *Presse Med.* 60:1456, 1952.

   First description of the technique. First employed in 1942 in the care of World War II battle casualties.

2. Borja, A. R. Current status of infraclavicular subclavian vein catheterization. *Ann. Thorac. Surg.* 13:615, 1972.

   Excellent review of the technique and especially of its complications.

3. Borja, A. R., and Hinshaw, J. R. A safe way to perform infraclavicular subclavian vein catheterization. *Surg. Gynecol. Obstet.* 130:673, 1970.

   Good description of the anatomy with a clear drawing.

4. Keeri-Szanto, M. The subclavian vein, a constant and convenient intravenous injection site. *Arch. Surg.* 72:179, 1956.

   One of the earliest English language descriptions of the anatomy of the cannulation technique.

5. Wilson, J. N., Grow, J. B., DeMong, C. V., et al. Central venous pressure in optimal blood volume to maintenance. *Arch. Surg.* 85:563, 1962.

   Early and complete description of the method and indications.

4.
Internal Jugular Vein Cannulation

Method of
Thomas J. Vander Salm

INDICATIONS (same as for subclavian vein cannulation, Chapter 3)

Central venous pressure measurement

Hyperalimentation

Vasopressor administration

Emergency IV route

Note: Because of fewer complications, this method is preferred to subclavian vein cannulation.

EQUIPMENT (see Appendix for sample kit)

Skin prep

   Sterile sponges

   Alcohol-acetone solution

   Povidone-iodine solution

Sterile field

   Mask, gown, gloves

   Towels

   Half sheet

   Towel clips

Local anesthetic

   Plastic syringe, 3-ml with 22-gauge × 1½-inch needle

   Lidocaine 1%, 5 ml

   For alternative technique: 22-gauge, 3-inch spinal needle

Cannulation equipment

    Plastic syringe (non-Luer-Lok), 3-ml

    Subclavian Jugular Catheter Set (Deseret), 14-gauge

    or

    Intracath (Deseret), 14-gauge, 12-inch

    Injectable saline, 30 ml

    Scissors, suture

    3-0 skin suture

Dressing

    Povidone-iodine ointment

    Sponges

    Tincture of benzoin

    Adhesive tape

      1-inch

      3-inch

Infusion

    Intravenous solution, tubing, and stand

Figure 1

POSITION (same as for subclavian vein cannulation)

Supine

10–20 degrees Trendelenburg

Head turned to opposite side

Roll under shoulders

MIDNECK TECHNIQUE

Figure 1

1. Prep and drape neck

Figure 2

    Identify anatomical landmarks.

2. Use mask, gown, and gloves

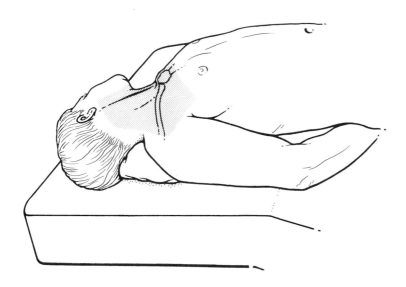

Figure 1
Position, prep, and drape.

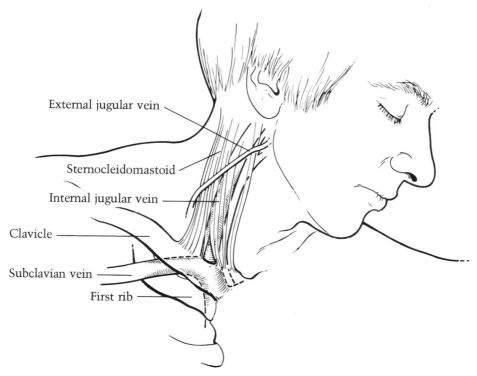

External jugular vein

Sternocleidomastoid

Internal jugular vein

Clavicle

Subclavian vein

First rib

Figure 2
Anatomical landmarks.

Figure 3

3. Infiltrate local anesthetic

Insert needle next to junction of posterior border of sternocleidomastoid muscle and external jugular vein (or 3 fingerbreadths above clavicle at posterior border of sternocleidomastoid muscle).

Aim for suprasternal notch.

Aspirate intermittently as needle advances.

Free return of venous blood confirms location of internal jugular vein.

Figure 4

4. Insert cannulation (Intracath) needle (on non-Luer-Lok syringe) into same puncture site; aim for suprasternal notch

5. Advance needle, aspirating gently; when venous blood returns freely, remove syringe and slide cannula through needle into internal jugular vein

Confirm free return of venous blood during a 360-degree axial rotation of the needle.

Pulsatile resistance indicates carotid artery. Withdraw needle, repeat step 4.

Occlude needle hub with finger to prevent bleeding or air entrainment while preparing to insert cannula.

Maintain Trendelenburg position sufficiently steep to cause venous efflux from open needle.

Advance cannula into superior vena cava (about 15 cm in adults).

Do not advance cannula if resistance is encountered.

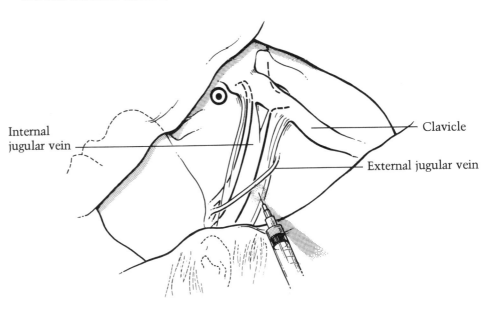

Figure 3
Infiltrate local anesthetic.

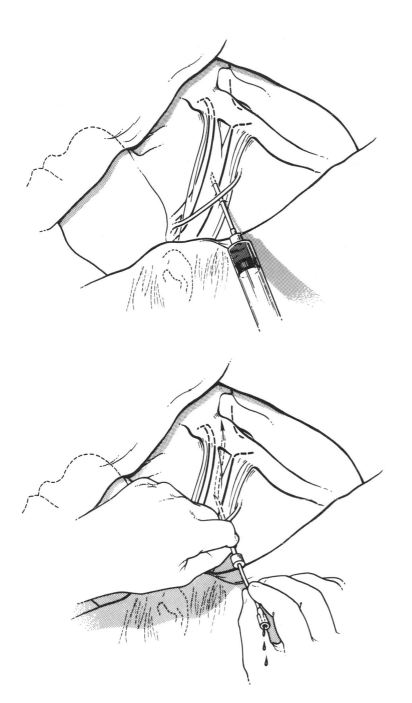

Figure 4
Insert cannulation needle.
Aim for suprasternal
notch, aspirate.

Figure 5
When venous blood re-
turns freely, remove
syringe and slide cannula
through needle into internal jugular vein.

ALTERNATIVE NEEDLE INSERTION TECHNIQUE (obviates searching for vein with larger needle)

Figure 6A

3A. Infiltrate local anesthetic with spinal needle threaded through Intracath needle

Figure 6B

4A. With free return of venous blood, slide Intracath needle into vein. Withdraw spinal needle

Figures 4, 5

5A. Transfer syringe to Intracath needle; confirm return of venous blood; slide cannula into vein

Figure 7

6. Withdraw needle; lock cannula and needle hubs together

With Subclavian Jugular Catheter, slide needle off cannula and screw hub onto cannula.

With Intracath, apply needle guard.

7. Aspirate, then flush cannula with saline-filled syringe

Aspirate to confirm free flow of blood.

Flush to prevent blood clotting in cannula.

Figure 7

8. Suture cannula to skin

Reaspirate and flush to confirm patency.

Figure 8

9. Apply dressing

Curve cannula onto chest so that major portion of dressing is off the neck for patient comfort.

Apply povidone-iodine ointment to puncture site.

Apply tincture of benzoin to surrounding skin.

Apply sterile dressing, securely taped.

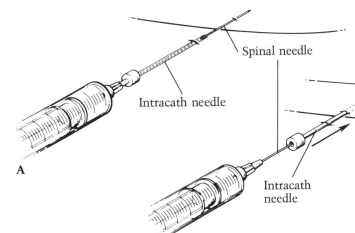

Figure 6A
Alternative method of finding vein: infiltrate local anesthetic with spinal needle threaded through Intracath needle.

Figure 6B
With free return of venous blood, slide Intracath needle into vein. Withdraw spinal needle.

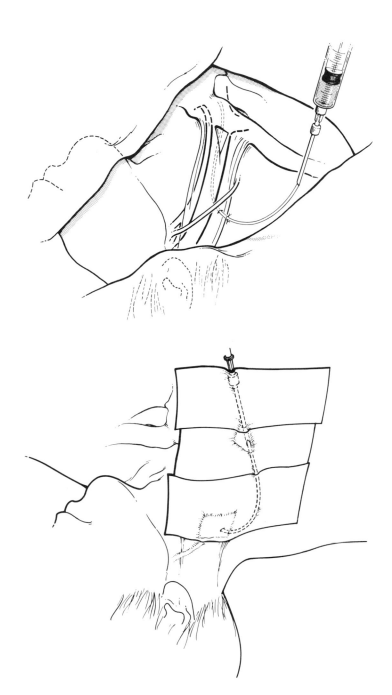

Figure 7
Withdraw needle; lock
cannula and needle hubs
together. Suture cannula to
skin.

Figure 8
Apply dressing.

10. **Begin infusion**

   Remove syringe.

   Attach cannula to intravenous tubing.

11. **Return bed to head-up position; assess for respiratory difficulty**

12. **Obtain chest x-ray**

   Rule out hemothorax or pneumothorax.

   Confirm cannula position in superior vena cava.

SUPRACLAVICULAR TECHNIQUE

1, 2. **Same as midneck technique**

   3. **Infiltrate with local anesthetic**

   Insert needle in center of triangle formed by clavicle and clavicular and sternal heads of sternocleidomastoid muscle.

   Advance needle in sagittal plane, aiming caudally and 30 degrees posteriorly.

   Aspirate intermittently.

   Free return of venous blood confirms location of internal jugular vein.

4–12. **Proceed as in midneck technique.**

COMPLICATIONS

Hematoma

Etiology

   Venous or arterial bleeding.

Prevention

   Do not advance needle if pulsations are felt through it.

   Adhere to proper line of needle advancement.

   Insert cannula gently; too much force will push it through wall of vein.

   Raise head of bed at completion to reduce venous pressure.

Air embolism

Etiology

   Air entrained through open cannula or needle due to insufficient internal jugular venous pressure.

Prevention

   Maintain sufficiently steep Trendelenburg position.

   Open cannula or needle to atmosphere only briefly.

   Maintain all connections in lines airtight.

Figure 9

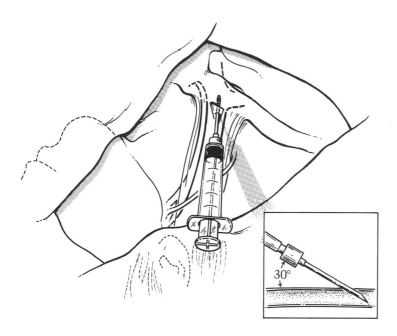

Figure 9
Supraclavicular approach.

Thoracic duct fistula

Etiology

Laceration of the thoracic duct.

Prevention

Use supraclavicular technique on right side only.

Pneumothorax or hemothorax

Etiology

Same as with subclavian vein cannulation (Chapter 3) but much less common; hence the advantage of the internal jugular technique.

Prevention

Same as with subclavian vein cannulation.

Vein thrombosis, infection, catheter embolism, myocardial puncture, hydromediastinum or hydrothorax.

Etiology

Same as with subclavian vein cannulation.

Prevention

Same as with subclavian vein cannulation.

CARE OF INTERNAL JUGULAR CANNULA

Same as for subclavian vein cannulation, Chapter 3.

SELECTED BIBLIOGRAPHY

1. Civetta, J. M., Gabel, J. C., and Gemer, M. Internal jugular vein puncture with a margin of safety. *Anesthesiology* 36:622, 1972.

   Description of method of locating vein with spinal needle threaded through the Intracath needle.

2. Daily, P. O., Griepp, R. B., and Shumway, N. E. Percutaneous internal jugular vein cannulation. *Arch. Surg.* 101:534, 1970.

   Good description of the alternative (supraclavicular) technique.

3. Jernigan, W. R., et al. Use of the internal jugular vein for placement of central venous catheter. *Surg. Gynecol. Obstet.* 130:520, 1970.

   Early description of the method described here.

5.
Internal Jugular Vein Cutdown

Method of
Thomas J. Vander Salm

INDICATIONS

Central venous pressure measurement

Hyperalimentation

Vasopressor administration

(Primarily in children and infants, or where percutaneous method otherwise not feasible)

EQUIPMENT (see Appendix for sample kit)

Skin prep

    Sterile sponges

    Alcohol-acetone solution

    Povidone-iodine solution

    Petrolatum gauze, 1-inch wide

Sterile field

    Mask, gown, gloves

    Towels, 4

    Towel clips, 4

Local anesthetic

    Syringe, 2-ml

    Needles

        25-gauge × ⅝-inch

        22-gauge × 1½-inch

    Lidocaine 1%, 10 ml

Cutdown equipment

    Sterile sponges

    Syringes

        10-ml

        2-ml

    Knife handle, #3

    Scalpel blades

        #11

        #15

    Retractors

        Self-retaining

        Rake, 2

    Forceps

        Fine-toothed

        Smooth

Scissors

   Suture

   Metzenbaum

   Curved iris

Clamps

   5, curved and straight mosquito

Needle holder

Cutdown catheter assortment, Silastic preferred, 16-, 18-, 20-gauge

Needle, 14-gauge × 1½-inch

Ligatures, 3-0 silk

Vascular suture, 5-0

Sutures

   Skin

   Subcutaneous

Injectable saline

Dressing

   Povidone-iodine ointment

   Sponges

   Tincture of benzoin

   Adhesive tape, 1-inch

Infusion

   Intravenous solution, tubing, and stand

Figure 1

POSITION

Supine

Head turned to opposite side

TECHNIQUE

Figure 1

1. Use mask, gown, and gloves

2. Prep and drape

From midline to occiput, including the ear in infants

Occlude auditory meatus with petrolatum gauze to exclude prep solutions from auditory canal.

3. Infiltrate local anesthetic

Figure 2

4. Incise skin, platysma, and subcutaneous tissue

Transverse incision

Anterior border sternocleidomastoid at junction of upper and middle thirds

Figure 3

5. Expose internal jugular and common facial veins

Retract sternocleidomastoid muscle laterally.

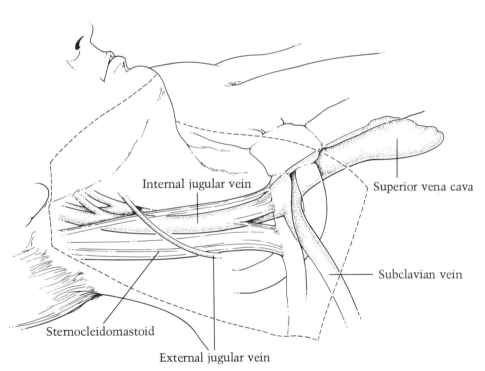

Internal jugular vein

Superior vena cava

Subclavian vein

Sternocleidomastoid

External jugular vein

Figure 1
Position, prep, and drape.

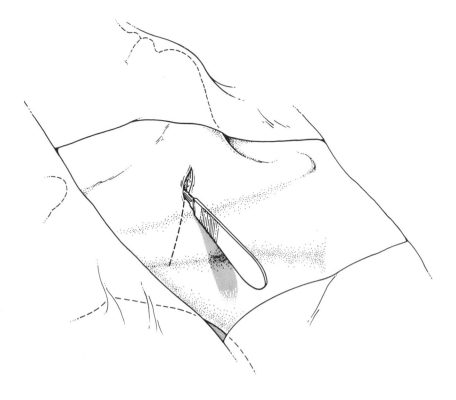

Figure 2
Incise skin, platysma, and
subcutaneous tissue.

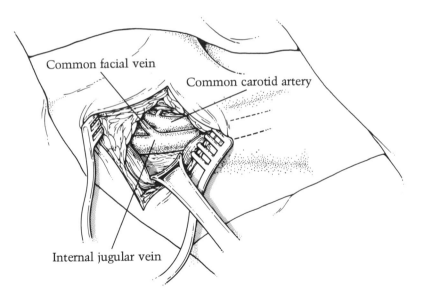

Common facial vein

Common carotid artery

Internal jugular vein

Figure 3
Expose internal jugular and
common facial veins.

6. Bring cannula through separate stab wound

Pass 14-gauge needle from incision, through sternocleidomastoid muscle, and out through skin (above mastoid process in infants) from inside out.

Pass cannula through needle from outside in.

Remove needle.

DIRECT CANNULATION WITHOUT LIGATION

7. Select appropriate size cannula

Figure 5

8. Place purse string suture on internal jugular vein

5-0 vascular suture

Superficial aspect of internal jugular vein

Purse string diameter slightly larger than that of cannula

9. Insert cannula

Make stab wound in center of purse string with needle slightly larger than cannula.

Pass cannula through stab wound; advance into superior vena cava.

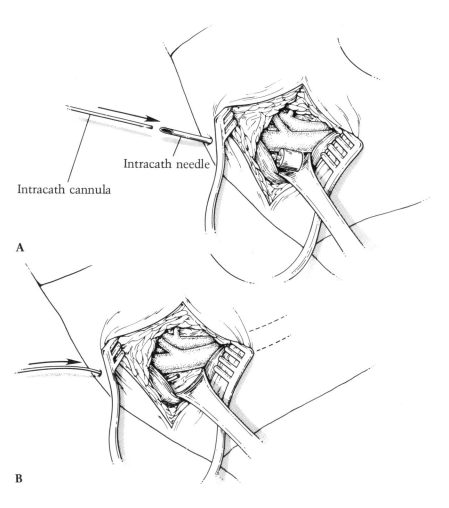

Intracath needle

Intracath cannula

A

Figure 4
Bring cannula through
separate stab wound.

B

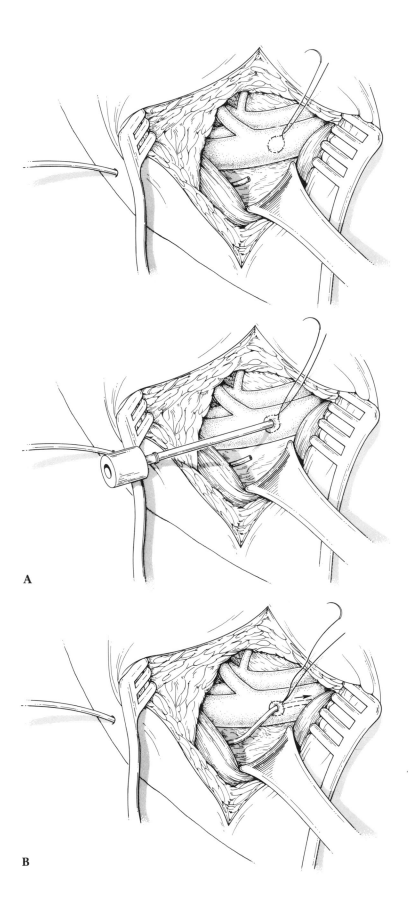

Figure 5
Place purse string suture
on internal jugular vein.

A

B

Figure 6
Insert cannula.

Figure 7

10. Flush cannula

Use saline-filled syringe.

Aspirate to confirm free flow of blood.

Flush to prevent clot formation.

Figure 8

11. Secure cannula

Tie purse string.

Reaspirate and flush to confirm patency.

Figure 9

12. Close incision

Separate layers for platysma and skin.

Suture cannula to skin at exit point.

Reconfirm cannula patency.

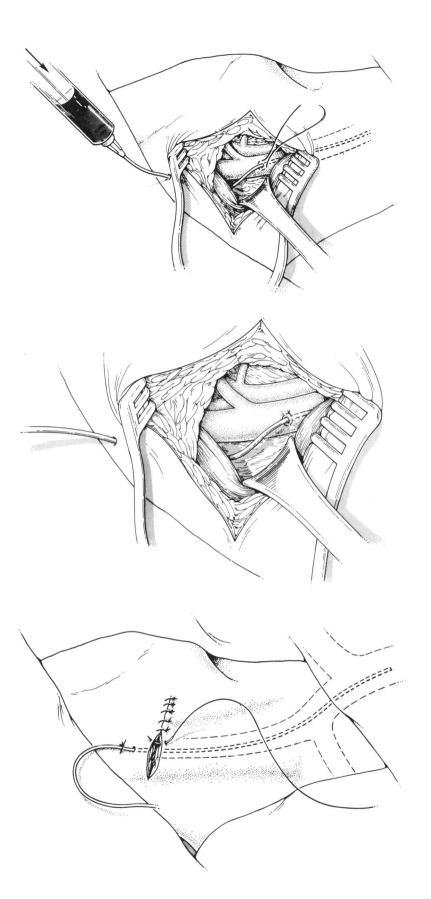

Figure 7
Flush cannula.

Figure 8
Secure cannula.

Figure 9
Close incision, suture
cannula.

Figure 10

13. Apply dressing

Apply povidone-iodine ointment to incision and stab wound.

Apply sterile dressing to each area.

Securely tape dressings and *cannula*.

14. Begin infusion

Remove syringe, attach intravenous tubing.

DIRECT CANNULATION WITH LIGATION

7–16. Perform on internal jugular vein as in venous cutdown, Chapter 2, steps 6–15

Thread cannula into superior vena cava about 15 cm.

Do not use unless contralateral vein is patent.

INDIRECT CANNULATION

Figure 11

7–16. Perform on common facial vein as in venous cutdown, steps 6–15

Thread cannula via common facial vein into internal jugular vein and thence into superior vena cava about 15 cm.

COMPLICATIONS

Same as for percutaneous method (Chapter 1), with same etiologies and prevention.

Complications due to blind cannulation (carotid artery puncture, thoracic duct fistula, and hemothorax or pneumothorax) are obviated, however.

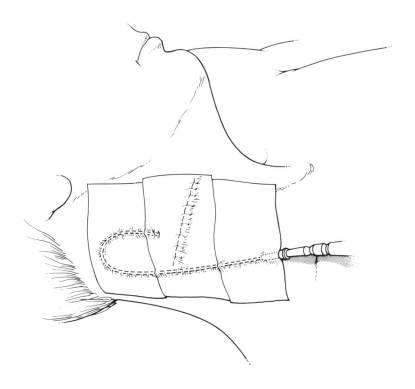

Figure 10
Apply dressing.

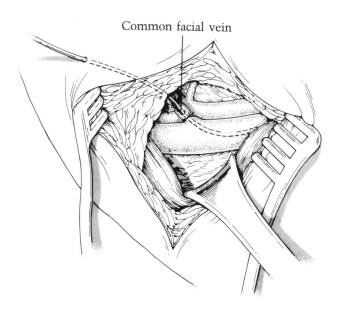

Common facial vein

Figure 11
Alternative cannulation
through common facial
vein.

SELECTED BIBLIOGRAPHY

1. Filler, R. M., Eraklis, A. J., Rubin, V. G., et al. Long-term total parenteral nutrition in infants. *N. Engl. J. Med.* 281:589, 1969.

   Description of technique of subcutaneous tunneling of the cannula.

2. Zumbro, G. L., Mullin, M. J., and Nelson, T. G. Catheter placement in infants needing total parenteral nutrition utilizing common facial vein. *Arch. Surg.* 102:71, 1971.

   Excellent description and drawings of the technique.

6.
Intravenous Regional Anesthesia

Method of Adrian S. Selwyn

INDICATIONS

Anesthesia for the hand, forearm, leg, or foot when local anesthesia is insufficient and less than 1–1½ hours is required

It is the method of choice for patients with full stomachs, respiratory or cardiovascular diseases, or any conditions in which general anesthesia may be hazardous.

CONTRAINDICATIONS

Extreme nervousness or psychological disturbance

Hypersensitivity to local anesthetic agents

Prolonged surgery (> 1½ hours)

Peripheral neurological disease (risk of nerve damage)

Peripheral vascular disease in the involved extremity

Local infections

EQUIPMENT (see Appendix for sample kit)

General

Blood pressure cuff

Intravenous line in noninvolved arm

Resuscitation equipment

Suction

Oxygen

Means of establishing airway and maintaining ventilation

Drugs for resuscitation

Tourniquet and exsanguination

Double cuff pneumatic tourniquet (single cuff adequate for short procedures)

Webril or Velband bandage

Rubber bandage (Esmarch or Martin)

Skin prep

Sterile sponges

Povidone-iodine solution

Intravenous cannulation

Butterfly needle, 21-gauge

or

Plastic cannula, 20-gauge (Angiocath or similar over-the-needle cannula)

Syringe, 10-ml

Needle, 18-gauge × 1½-inch

Injectable saline

Adhesive tape, 1-inch

Anesthetic administration

Syringe, 50-ml

Lidocaine ½%, 50 ml (*without epinephrine*)

POSITION

Supine

Involved extremity completely exposed

TECHNIQUE

1. **Check equipment**

   Resuscitation equipment

   Tourniquet

2. **Establish intravenous line in noninvolved arm**

3. **Measure blood pressure in noninvolved arm**

Figure 1

4. **Cannulate vein of involved extremity**

   Use distal vein (hand, wrist, or foot).

   Use butterfly needle or plastic cannula (see Chapter 1).

   Flush cannula/needle with saline to preserve patency.

Figure 2

5. **Apply tourniquet**

   Wrap upper portion of extremity with soft bandage (e.g., Webril), and apply tourniquet over this padding.

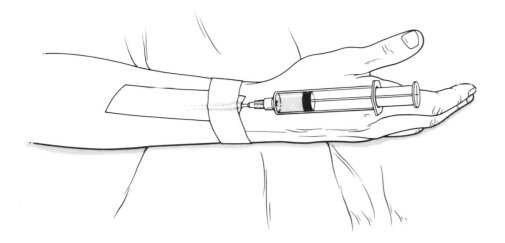

Figure 1
Cannulate vein of involved
extremity.

Tourniquet

Soft padding

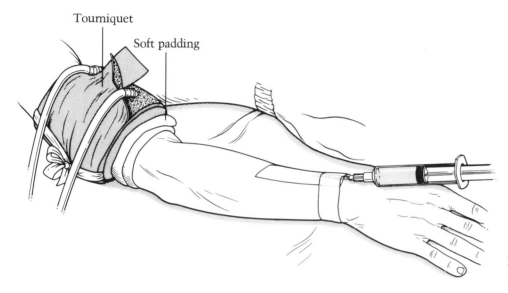

Figure 2
Apply tourniquet.

Figure 3

6. Exsanguinate limb

Remove syringe; replace occlusive plug in IV cannula.

Elevate extremity.

Wrap firmly from distal to proximal with rubber (Esmarch) bandage.

Overlap each turn one-half width of bandage.

If presence of limb trauma makes wrapping painful, elevate limb and compress arterial inflow for 5 minutes to achieve exsanguination.

Figure 4

7. Inflate tourniquet

Inflate proximal (upper) cuff to well above systolic blood pressure

Usually 300 mm Hg in arms

Usually 500 mm Hg in legs

Ascertain that cuff remains inflated.

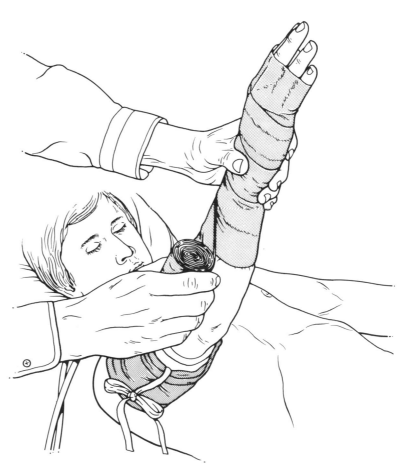

Figure 3
Exsanguinate limb.

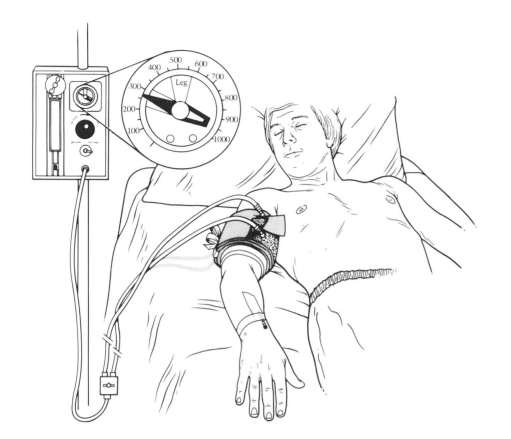

Figure 4
Inflate tourniquet.

8. Remove rubber (Esmarch) bandage

Good exsanguination manifest by diffuse pallor

Blotchy appearance indicates less complete exsanguination—dilution of anesthetic may result in patchy anesthesia.

Figure 5

9. Inject local anesthetic

Use previously placed needle/cannula.

Use lidocaine *without epinephrine*.

Concentration: 0.5% arm; 0.25% leg

Dose: about 3 mg/kg

Usual volume: 40–50 ml, arm; 80–100 ml, leg

(Volume as important as concentration)

Inject over several minutes; then remove needle/cannula.

10. Prepare for surgical procedure

Ascertain that cuff not leaking.

Anesthesia usually complete in 5 minutes

11. Tourniquet management

Tourniquet discomfort: onset about 20 minutes

Relieve by inflating distal cuff, then releasing proximal cuff when certain that distal cuff not leaking.

With single cuff tourniquet, prior infiltration of band of local anesthetic above cuff ameliorates pain.

To prevent large bolus of lidocaine being released systemically, do not release tourniquet within 20 minutes of anesthetic injection.

After operative procedure, release tourniquet.

Anesthesia disappears within a few minutes.

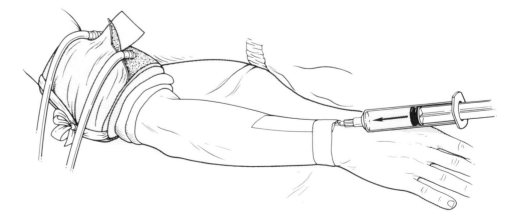

Figure 5
Inject local anesthetic.

COMPLICATIONS

Failure of anesthesia

Etiology

Inadequate exsanguination of extremity.

Prevention

Ascertain adequate exsanguination (diffuse pallor without mottling) before injection.

Short duration of anesthesia

Etiology

Tourniquet leaking—allows dilution of lidocaine.

Prevention

Check tourniquet for leaks before lidocaine injected.

Systemic toxic reactions

Etiology

Lidocaine allergy (rare).

Cuff leak or premature cuff deflation, causing systemic bolus of lidocaine. (After 20 minutes, lidocaine is fixed in tissues sufficiently to prevent sudden bolus.)

Prevention

Avoid technique in presence of lidocaine allergy.

Ascertain cuff integrity before injecting lidocaine.

Do not release cuff within 20 minutes of lidocaine injection.

TREATMENT OF TOXICITY

Circulatory depression

Trendelenburg position

IV fluids

Vasopressors if necessary

Face mask oxygen

Respiratory depression

Face mask oxygen

Artificial ventilation if necessary

Endotracheal intubation if necessary

CNS stimulation

If mild, face mask oxygen

If severe (tremors, convulsions), IV thiopental or Valium

SELECTED BIBLIOGRAPHY

1. Bier, A.   Über einen neuen Weg Lokalanästhesie an den Gliedmassen zu erzeugen. *Arch. Klin. Chir.* 86:1007, 1908.

   First description of this technique.

2. Knapp, R. B.   The physiological mechanism behind intravenous regional anesthesia. *Acta Anaesthesiol. Scand. [Suppl.]* XIII, 1966.

   Physiological basis for the method.

3. Solomon, L., and Berkowitz, T.   Intravenous regional anesthesia. A simple method of anesthesia for limb surgery. *S. Afr. Med. J.* 39:844, 1965.

   Good description of the technique.

7.
Inferior Vena Caval Umbrella Filter

Method of
Thomas J. Vander Salm

INDICATIONS

Alternative to open interruption of inferior vena cava as a means of prevention of
pulmonary emboli

EQUIPMENT (see Appendix for sample kit)

X-ray

Fluoroscope and table

Skin prep

Sterile sponges

Alcohol-acetone solution

Povidone-iodine solution

Sterile field

Mask, gown, gloves

Towels, 4

Towel clips, 4

Large drapes, 4

or

Laparotomy sheet

Local anesthetic

   Syringe, 5-ml

   Needles

      25-gauge × ⅝-inch

      22-gauge × 1½-inch

   Lidocaine 1%, 20 ml

Procedure

   Mobin-Uddin sterile catheter assembly

   Sterile sponges

   Solution bowl

   Knife handle, #3

   Scalpel blades

      #10

      #11

   Retractors

      Self-retaining (Weitläner)

      Right-angle, 2

   Clamps

      5, curved or straight

   Scissors

      Suture

      Metzenbaum

      30-degree Potts

   Forceps

      Smooth, 2

      Toothed, 2

Vascular tourniquets, 2 (umbilical tape to thread through 8–10-cm length of 14 Fr. rubber tubing via Rummel obturator)

Needle holders

    1 vascular

    1 standard

Ligatures

    3-0 silk

    4-0 silk

Sutures

    5-0 vascular

    4-0 silk

    Skin

Dressing

    Sterile sponges

    Tincture of benzoin

    Adhesive tape, 1-inch

Figure 1

POSITION

Supine, on fluoroscopy table

Head turned to left

Roll under shoulders

TECHNIQUE

Obtain angiogram of inferior vena cava and renal veins.

1. **Use mask, gown, and gloves**

Figure 1

2. **Prep and drape**

   Right neck

   Supraclavicular area from ear to upper sternum

Figure 2A

3. **Assemble Mobin-Uddin apparatus**

Figure 2B

   Loosen stylette pin vise, slide back on stylette 5–6 cm away from Luer-Lok hub, and retighten.

Figure 2C

   Advance stylette until stylette pin vise encounters Luer-Lok hub.

Figure 2D

   Screw umbrella on distal end of stylette; unscrew one-half turn.

   Lubricate umbrella with water-soluble lubricant.

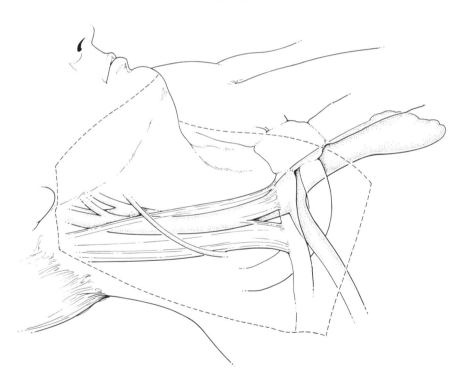

Figure 1
Position, prep, and drape.

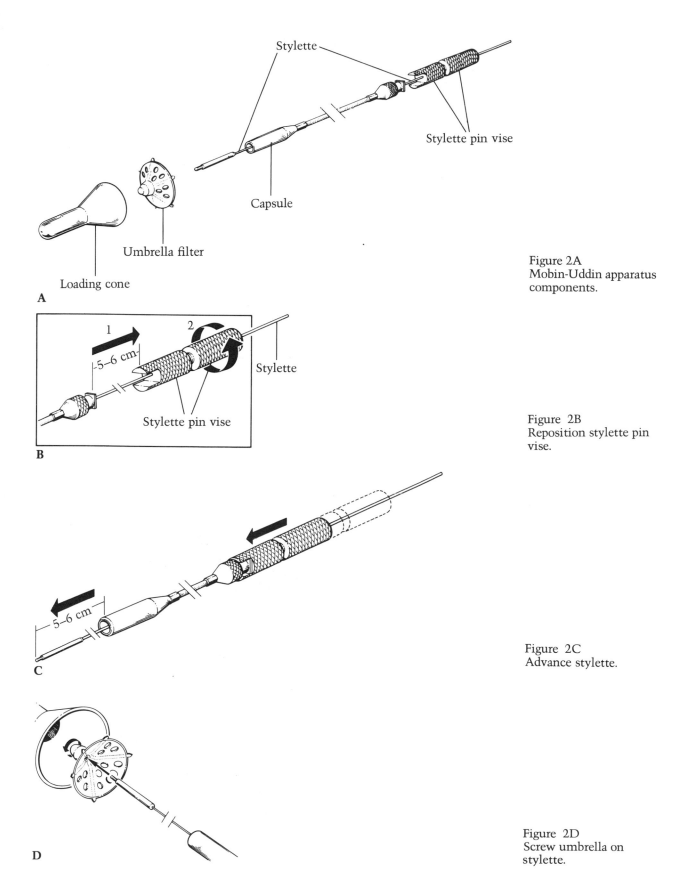

Stylette

Stylette pin vise

Capsule

Umbrella filter

Loading cone

A

Figure 2A
Mobin-Uddin apparatus
components.

1

2

5–6 cm

Stylette

Stylette pin vise

B

Figure 2B
Reposition stylette pin
vise.

5–6 cm

C

Figure 2C
Advance stylette.

D

Figure 2D
Screw umbrella on
stylette.

Figure 2E	Collapse umbrella into loading cone.
Figure 2F, G	Advance capsule into loading cone and pull stylette back to transfer umbrella into capsule.
	Advance stylette ejecting umbrella from capsule to test function; then reload as above.
Figure 2H	Loosen stylette pin vise, slide forward on stylette until it encounters Luer-Lok hub, and retighten (prevents accidental ejection or unscrewing of umbrella).

4. Infiltrate local anesthetic

Figure 3   **5. Incise skin, subcutaneous tissue, and platysma**

Transverse incision

Midportion of sternocleidomastoid, anterior border

Figure 4   **6. Isolate internal jugular vein**

Retract sternocleidomastoid muscle laterally.

Expose vein circumferentially.

Encircle and occlude vein with two vascular tourniquets, 3 cm apart.

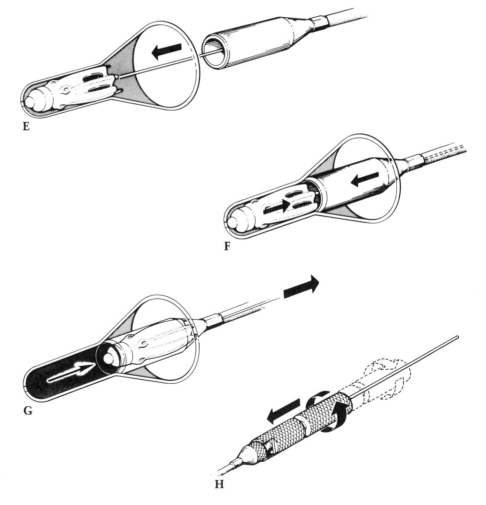

Figure 2E
Collapse umbrella into
loading cone.

Figure 2F, G
Load umbrella into cap-
sule.

Figure 2H
Reposition stylette pin
vise to prevent accidental
ejection.

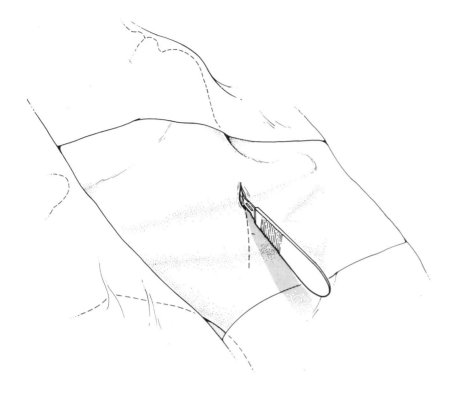

Figure 3
Incise skin, subcutaneous
tissue, and platysma.

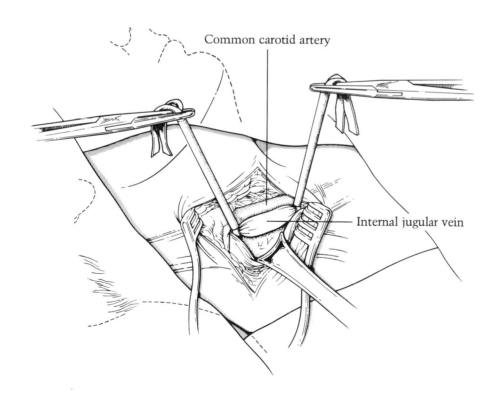

Common carotid artery

Internal jugular vein

Figure 4
Isolate internal jugular
vein.

7. Make venotomy

Longitudinal, 1 cm long

Figure 5

8. Insert capsule with umbrella

Momentarily release caudal tourniquet.

Pass capsule into vein—Trendelenburg position obviates air embolism.

Resecure caudal tourniquet over cannula.

Figure 6

9. Position capsule under fluoroscopic control

Advance to bifurcation of IVC (located from previous venogram).

Pull back until caudal end of capsule lies 1–2 cm below lowest renal vein (again determined from previous venogram).

Figure 7

10. Eject umbrella

Reposition stylette pin vise 4 cm from catheter.

Advance stylette, ejecting umbrella.

Use gentle traction on stylette to confirm fixed position in IVC and to seat spokes of umbrella.

Unscrew stylette from umbrella, continuing gentle traction.

Withdraw assembly, leaving umbrella in IVC.

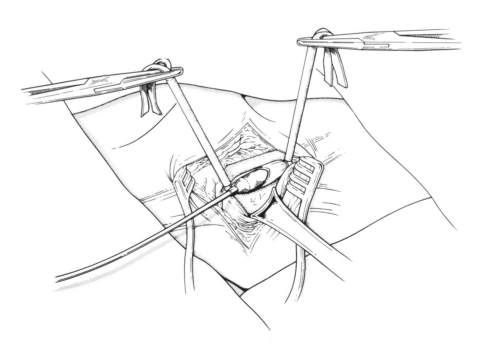

Figure 5
Insert capsule with
umbrella.

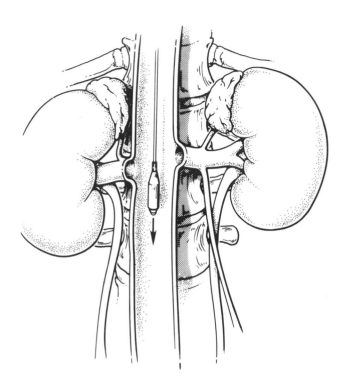

Figure 6
Position capsule under
fluoroscopic control.

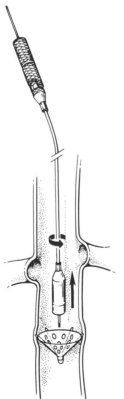

Figure 7
Eject umbrella.

Figure 8

11. Repair vein

Use running vascular suture.

Release tourniquets.

12. Close wound

Use separate layers for platysma and skin.

13. Apply dressing

Note: See reference [3] for description of the Greenfield vena caval filter. This filter may prove to be superior to the Mobin-Uddin filter, although follow-up on it at this time is shorter.

POSTOPERATIVE CARE

Heparin

Stop for 12 hours, then resume if no contraindications.

Leg support

Elevate legs when in bed.

Apply elastic leg support when ambulating.

COMPLICATIONS

Air embolism

Etiology

Air drawn in through venotomy secondary to negative internal jugular pressure.

Prevention

Increase internal jugular pressure with Trendelenburg position while cannula is inserted.

Cardiac arrhythmias

Etiology

Sinus node trauma as capsule passes through right atrium.

Prevention

Pass capsule into IVC atraumatically. If arrhythmias persist, withdraw into SVC until normal rhythm returns.

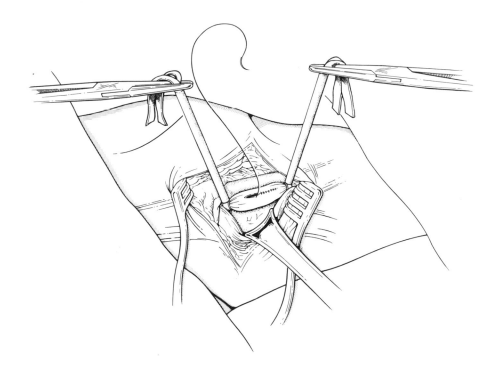

Figure 8
Repair vein.

Umbrella malposition

Etiology

Inadequate knowledge of venous anatomy, leading to placement above renal veins, in a renal vein, or in a common iliac vein.

Prevention

Use preoperative angiogram and bony landmarks to place umbrella correctly.

Advance capsule first to vena caval bifurcation, thus ensuring against deviation of capsule into a renal vein.

Failure of umbrella to open

Etiology

Incorrect loading.

Sticking of umbrella components to themselves or against vena cava.

Prevention

Check umbrella ejection before inserting.

If umbrella fails to open fully, advance capsule against concave side of umbrella while holding stylette fixed. This forces umbrella open.

Migration or embolization of umbrella

Etiology

Umbrella too small for vein or placement too high in vena cava.

Prevention

Use preoperative angiogram to choose proper placement and size of umbrella—the 28-mm size is usually used.

Retroperitoneal hemorrhage

Etiology

Laceration of inferior vena cava by umbrella.

Since umbrella spokes are specifically designed to penetrate into IVC wall, this is to some extent unavoidable.

Prevention (of large tears)

Avoid forceful traction on umbrella when it is seated into IVC.

Recurrent pulmonary embolization

Etiology

Malposition of umbrella in vessel other than IVC.

Prevention

Prevent as for malposition.

Etiology

Embolus source above the umbrella.

Prevention

Use preoperative venogram to rule out proximal source of emboli.

Etiology

Embolization from other limb of double vena cava.

Prevention

Determine presence of double IVC from angiogram. If present, insert an umbrella in each limb.

Etiology

Embolization from ovarian veins.

Prevention

Use open ligation if embolization from ovarian vein suspected in the presence of pelvic sepsis.

Chronic edema of legs

Etiology

Iliofemoral thrombophlebitis.

Total occlusion of IVC below umbrella occurs in about 70% of cases but alone does not account for chronic stasis changes—phlebitis also is necessarily present.

Prevention

Elevate legs when the patient is supine, and give effective elastic stocking support when ambulatory during collateral vein development.

SELECTED BIBLIOGRAPHY

1. Edwards Laboratories. Mobin-Uddin Vena Cava Umbrella Filters. Information brochure, January, 1974.

   Excellent description of techniques and complications.

2. Fullen, W. D., McDonough, J. J., and Altmeier, W. A. Clinical experience with vena caval filters. *Arch. Surg.* 106:582, 1973.

   Good emphasis of important points of insertion.

3. Greenfield, L. J., Zocco, J., Wilk, J., et al. Clinical experience with the Kim-Ray Greenfield vena caval filter. *Ann. Surg.* 185:692, 1977.

   Description of use and results of an alternative vena caval filter.

4. McConnell, D., Mulder, D., and Buckberg, G. The placement of vena caval umbrella filters. The value of phlebography. *Arch. Surg.* 108:789, 1974.

   Points out the pitfalls avoidable by phlebography.

5. Mobin-Uddin, K., Callard, G. M., Bolooki, H., et al. Transvenous caval interruption with umbrella filter. *N. Engl. J. Med.* 286:55, 1972.

   Follow-up on 100 patients. Complications reviewed, especially those of caval occlusion, chronic stasis (none present), and thrombophlebitis.

6. Mobin-Uddin, K., McLean, R., Bolooki, H., et al. Caval interruption for prevention of pulmonary embolism. Long-term results of a new method. *Arch. Surg.* 99:711, 1969.

   Good description of the technique of insertion.

7. Mobin-Uddin, K., Smith, P. E., Martinez, L. O., et al. A vena caval filter for the prevention of pulmonary embolus. *Surg. Forum* 18:208, 1967.

   Initial description of the filter.

8.
Arterial Puncture

Method of
Thomas J. Vander Salm

INDICATIONS

Obtaining arterial blood—most commonly, to determine PO_2, PCO_2, and pH

EQUIPMENT (see Appendix for sample kit)

Positioning

Armboard

Nonsterile towel

Adhesive tape, 1-inch

Skin prep

Povidone-iodine solution

Sterile sponges

Procedure

Glass syringe, 3-ml

Needles

20-gauge $\times$ 1½-inch

23-gauge $\times$ ⅝-inch

Heparin ampule, 1-ml, 1000 units/ml

Syringe cap

Plastic bag

Crushed ice

POSITION

Supine

Arteries commonly used are radial, common femoral, and brachial, in descending order of preference.

Figure 1   For radial artery, dorsiflex wrist over towel.

TECHNIQUE

Figure 1
1. **Prep selected site**

2. **Give local anesthetic (optional)**

3. **Wet syringe with heparin**

   Draw heparin into syringe through 20-gauge needle, wetting all inner surfaces.

   Replace 20-gauge needle with 23-gauge needle.

   Eject air and excess heparin.

   Leave needle and dead space filled with heparin.

Figure 2
4. **Insert needle through skin**

   Palpate artery with index finger.

   Thrust needle through skin at 60-degree angle.

   Slowly advance needle toward artery.

Figure 3
5. **Puncture artery, obtain blood**

   Arterial pulsation often palpable as transmitted by syringe when needle contacts artery.

   Confirm arterial puncture: pulsatile blood fills syringe.

   Note: Do not aspirate blood; allow syringe to fill by arterial pressure.

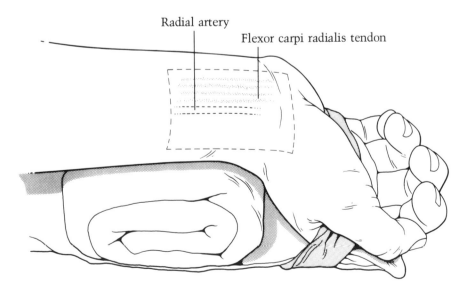

Radial artery

Flexor carpi radialis tendon

Figure 1
Position and prep.

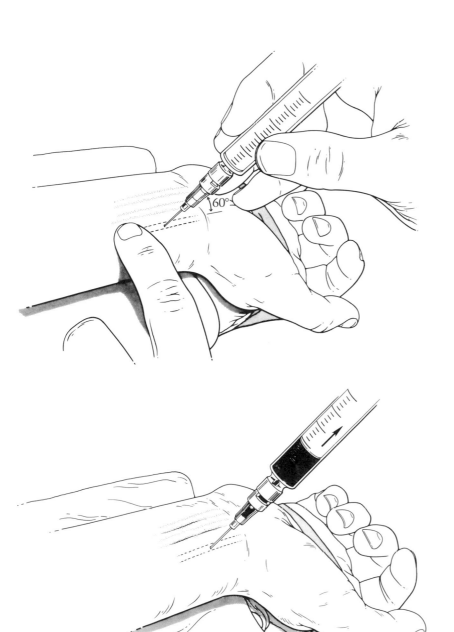

Figure 2
Insert needle through skin.

Figure 3
Puncture artery, obtain blood.

6. Withdraw needle and syringe

Apply firm, even pressure to puncture site for 5 minutes.

Avoid occluding artery: not necessary in order to stop bleeding from puncture site.

7. Send sample for analysis

Remove needle from syringe, eject any bubbles, and cap syringe.

Place syringe in ice to reduce red cell metabolism.

COMPLICATIONS

Local bleeding

Etiology

Pressure applied to puncture site for insufficient time.

Prevention

Apply pressure for full 5 minutes.

Venous admixture of blood

Etiology

Drawing venous blood into system by aspirating.

Prevention

Never aspirate blood; allow it to flow into syringe under arterial pressure.

Use short bevel needle so that tip of bevel will not project beyond lumen of artery.

Air admixture of blood

Etiology

Aspiration, causing air to leak in through syringe–needle connections.

Incomplete emptying of air from syringe before starting.

Prevention

Do not aspirate blood.

Eject all air from syringe before arterial puncture.

Distal ischemia

Etiology

Excessive arterial trauma with thrombosis.

Prevention

Use narrow-gauge needle.

Do not puncture same arterial site numerous consecutive times: rotate sites.

Avoid brachial artery puncture if possible; this site carries an increased incidence of ischemic complications.

SELECTED BIBLIOGRAPHY

1. Mathieu, A., Dalton, B., Fischer, J. E., et al. Expanding aneurysm of the radial artery after frequent puncture. *Anesthesiology* 38:401, 1973.

   Description of a rare complication.

2. Petty, T. L., Bigelow, B., and Levine, B. E. The simplicity and safety of arterial puncture. *J.A.M.A.* 195:693, 1966.

   Good description of the technique.

9.
Arterial Cannula Insertion, Percutaneous

Method of Thomas J. Vander Salm

INDICATIONS

Arterial pressure monitoring

Repeated arterial blood sampling

Cardiac output measurement by dye-dilution technique

EQUIPMENT (see Appendix for sample kit)

Positioning

Armboard

Folded towel

Adhesive tape, 1-inch

Skin prep

Sterile sponges

Alcohol-acetone solution

Povidone-iodine solution

Sterile field

Towel

Local anesthetic

Syringe, 2-ml

Needle, 25-gauge × ⅝-inch

Lidocaine 1%, 1-ml ampule

Arterial cannulation

    Syringe, 10-ml

    Angiocath, 18-gauge, or Medicut cannula, 18-gauge

    Stopcock, 3-way

    Heparin, 1 ml of 1000 units/ml

    Injectable saline, 30-ml vial

Dressing

    Povidone-iodine ointment

    Sterile sponges

    Tincture of benzoin

    Adhesive tape, 1-inch

Pressure monitoring

    Arterial pressure transducer

    Pressure tubing

    Calibrated oscilloscope

CONFIRM ADEQUATE COLLATERAL CIRCULATION

Confirm presence of radial and ulnar pulses.

Use Allen test.

Figure 1A

Figure 1B

Simultaneously occlude radial and ulnar arteries with thumbs. Patient exsanguinates hand by repeated forced clenching, then partially opens hand. When hand blanched, release compression of one artery. Normal color should return within 3–5 seconds. Repeat with other artery.

If adequate radial *and* ulnar circulation not confirmed, do not cannulate either artery.

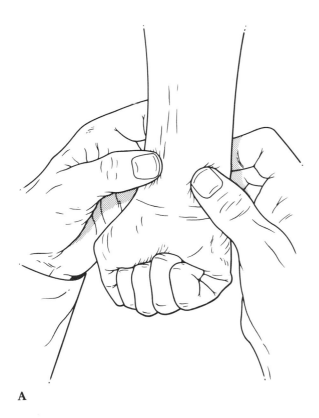

A

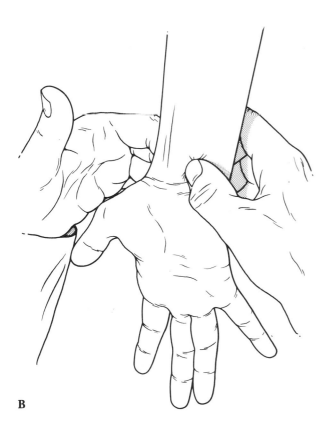

B

Figure 1
Confirm adequate collateral circulation. A. Occlude radial and ulnar arteries. B. Release radial artery to test its patency; repeat test for ulnar artery.

POSITION

Figure 2

For radial artery cannulation: supine, arm abducted, forearm supinated

Arteries used less frequently (brachial, dorsalis pedis, common femoral): supine, artery positioned uppermost

TECHNIQUE (for radial artery; others are similar)

Figure 2

1. **Dorsiflex wrist**

   Place folded towel between wrist and armboard.

   Tape palm to maintain position.

Figure 2

2. **Prep, drape wrist**

3. **Infiltrate local anesthetic**

   Do not obscure artery by injecting excessive amount.

4. **Fill syringe**

   10 ml heparinized saline (500 units heparin per 10 ml)

   Attach stopcock to syringe.

Figure 3

5. **Insert Angiocath through skin**

   45-degree angle with axis of artery

Figure 4

6. **Cannulate artery**

   Transfix artery

   Arterial flow through needle confirms entry.

   Advance until artery transfixed by needle and cannula.

   Remove needle, leaving cannula in place.

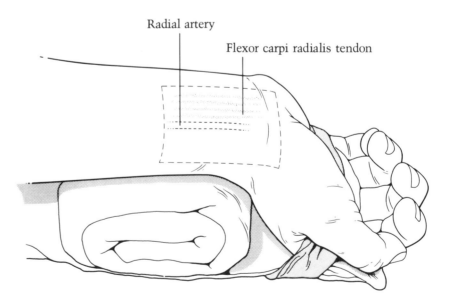

Figure 2
Dorsiflex wrist, prep, and drape.

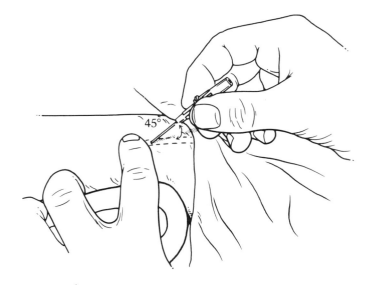

Figure 3
Insert Angiocath through skin.

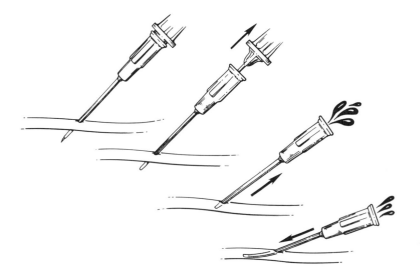

Figure 4
Cannulate artery.

Place cannula in artery

Slowly withdraw cannula until arterial blood spurts out.

Quickly but gently advance cannula up artery.

Vigorous arterial back bleeding confirms proper position.

Figure 5

6A. Cannulate artery, alternative technique

Puncture front wall of artery—arterial flow through needle confirms entry.

Advance needle/cannula up artery until cannula tip in artery.

Remove needle and advance cannula.

Vigorous arterial back bleeding continues through this step.

Note: This technique avoids hole in back wall of artery; some find it more difficult, however.

7. Control bleeding

Apply pressure over artery at tip of cannula.

Figure 6

8. Flush cannula

Attach syringe with stopcock.

Aspirate to confirm good flow.

Flush with heparinized saline to prevent clot formation.

Close stopcock to cannula; remove syringe from stopcock.

Figure 7

9. Apply dressing

Apply tincture of benzoin to skin.

Apply povidone-iodine ointment to puncture site.

Securely tape sterile dressing, *cannula,* and *stopcock.*

10. Attach transducer tubing

Tape or clip all connections securely.

11. Apply pressure to site for 5 minutes to stop bleeding

12. Reapply armboard

Release tape on palm.

Remove towel.

Retape hand to armboard.

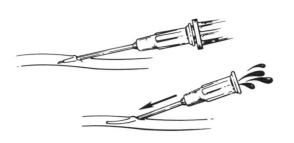

Figure 5
Cannulate artery (alternative technique).

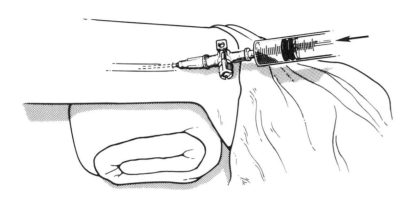

Figure 6
Flush cannula.

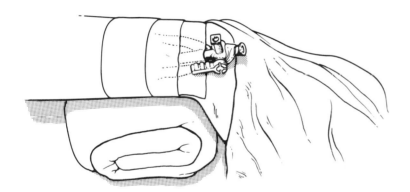

Figure 7
Apply dressing.

COMPLICATIONS

Finger ischemia

Etiology

> Diminished flow to hand.

> Usually seen in shock and/or with poor ulnar artery flow.

Prevention

> Cannulate radial artery only if ipsilateral ulnar artery has good flow as confirmed by Allen test.

> If shock or a low flow state exists, benefits from the procedure should be weighed against possible complications of ischemia.

Bleeding at puncture site

Etiology

> Inadequate application of local pressure.

Prevention

> Maintain local pressure over puncture site for full 5 minutes.

Bleeding from arterial line

Etiology

> Separation of components of system.

> Massive bleeding may result.

Prevention

> Tape or clip all couplings of system.

> Never leave patient unattended.

Retrograde arterial embolism

Etiology

> Retrograde flushing of cannula may embolize clots into cerebral circulation.

> Greater danger with smaller patients; even in adults, 3-ml boluses can reach cerebral circulation via retrograde flow.

Prevention

> Use volumes smaller than 3 ml (less in children) when flushing cannula, or use slow, continuous flushing to maintain patency.

SELECTED BIBLIOGRAPHY

1. Allen, E. V. Thromboangiitis obliterans; methods of diagnosis of chronic occlusive arterial lesions distal to the wrist with illustrative cases. *Am. J. Med. Sci.* 178:237, 1929.

   Description by Allen of the Allen test.

2. Barr, P. Percutaneous puncture of the radial artery with a multi-purpose Teflon catheter for indwelling use. *Acta Physiol. Scand.* 51:343, 1961.

   One of the first reports of arterial cannulation using the method described by Massa.

3. Evans, D., and Ozer, S. A simple method of arterial cannulation. *Can. Anaesth. Soc. J.* 17:181, 1970.

   Description of the transfixion technique.

4. Foti, P. R., and Moser, K. M. An effective, simple technique for indwelling arterial cannulation with Teflon. *Angiology* 20:439, 1969.

   Description of needle/cannula/stylette combination (Becton-Dickson) used with the transfixion technique.

5. Lowenstein, E., Little, J. W., III, and Lo, H. H. Prevention of cerebral embolization from flushing radial-artery cannulas. *N. Engl. J. Med.* 285:1414, 1971.

   Studies showing that injection in radial artery of boluses as small as 3 ml (average, 7 ml) were sufficient to cause cerebral embolization via retrograde flow in the arm.

6. Massa, D. J., Lundy, J. S., Faulconer, A., Jr., et al. A plastic needle. *Mayo Clin. Proc.* 25:413, 1950.

   One of the first reports of the needle in a cannula technique but used for venous cannulation.

7. Mortensen, J. D. Clinical sequelae from arterial needle puncture, cannulation and incision. *Circulation* 35:1118, 1967.

   A catalog of the many complications seen, especially with brachial artery puncture (when done for arteriography).

10.
Arterial Cannula Insertion, Cutdown

Method of
Thomas J. Vander Salm

INDICATIONS

Arterial pressure monitoring

Repeated arterial blood sampling

Cardiac output measurement by dye-dilution technique

When percutaneous method not feasible

EQUIPMENT (see Appendix for sample kit)

Positioning

Armboard

Folded towel

Adhesive tape, 1-inch

Skin prep

Sterile sponges

Acetone-alcohol solution

Povidone-iodine solution

Sterile field

Mask, gown, gloves

Towels, 4

Towel clips

Local anesthetic

Plastic syringe, 2-ml

Needle, 25-gauge × ⅝-inch

Lidocaine 1%, 10 ml

Cannula insertion

   Sterile sponges

   Knife handle, #3

   Scalpel blade, #15

   Scissors

     Curved iris

     Suture

   Forceps, fine-toothed

   Clamps, 2 curved mosquito

   Retractors

     1 small self-retaining

   Needle holder

   Ligatures, 3-0 silk

   Syringe, 10-ml plastic

   Angiocath, 18-gauge, or Medicut cannula, 18-gauge

   Stopcock, 3-way

   Heparin, 1 ml, 1000 units/ml

   Injectable saline, 30-ml vial

   Sutures, skin

Dressing

   Povidone-iodine ointment

   Sterile sponges

   Tincture of benzoin

   Adhesive tape, 1-inch

Pressure monitoring

   Arterial pressure transducer

   Pressure tubing

   Calibrated oscilloscope

CONFIRM ADEQUATE COLLATERAL CIRCULATION (see Chapter 9)

Confirm presence of radial and ulnar pulses.

Use Allen test.

Simultaneously occlude radial and ulnar arteries with thumbs. Have patient exsanguinate hand by repeated forced clenching, then partially open hand. When hand is blanched, release compression of one artery. Normal color should return within 3–5 seconds. Repeat with other artery.

If adequate radial *and* ulnar circulation not confirmed, do not cannulate either artery.

BELMONT COLLEGE LIBRARY

POSITION

Figure 1

Same as for percutaneous method, Chapter 9

TECHNIQUE (for radial artery; similar for other arteries)

Figure 1

1. Dorsiflex wrist

Place folded towel between wrist and armboard.

Tape palm to secure position.

Figure 1

2. Prep, drape wrist

3. Infiltrate local anesthetic

Transversely

Directly over most prominent pulse

Figure 2

4. Incise skin and subcutaneous tissue

Figure 3

5. Isolate artery

Use blunt dissection, deep to fascia; artery lies deeper than expected.

Free artery circumferentially.

Expose 1–2 cm of artery.

6. Fill syringe

Use 10 ml heparinized saline (500 units heparin/10 ml).

Attach stopcock.

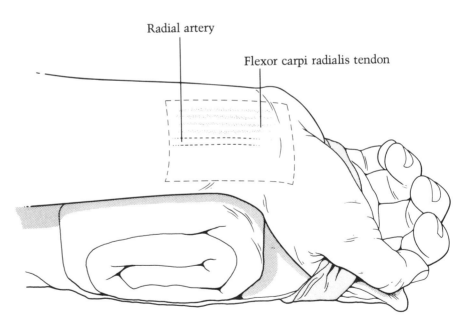

Radial artery

Flexor carpi radialis tendon

Figure 1
Dorsiflex wrist, prep, and drape.

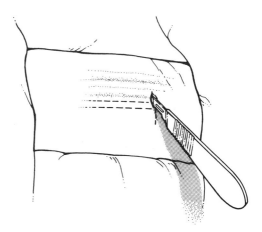

Figure 2
Incise skin and subcutaneous tissue.

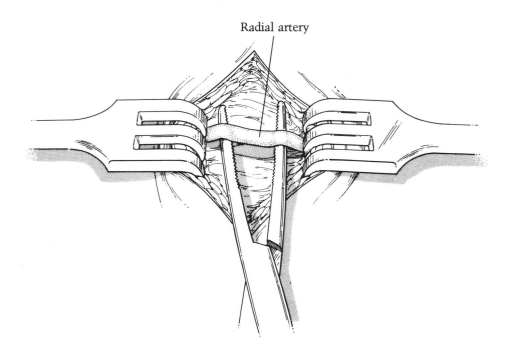

Radial artery

Figure 3
Isolate artery.

7. **Cannulate artery**

   Figure 4

   Use Angiocath.

   Puncture artery proximal to elevating clamp.

   Slide needle/cannula into artery until cannula tip lies in artery.

   Figure 5

   Remove needle and advance cannula.

   Vigorous arterial back bleeding continues during this step.

   Figure 6

8. **Flush cannula**

   Attach syringe with stopcock.

   Aspirate to confirm good flow.

   Flush with heparinized saline to prevent clot formation.

   Close stopcock to cannula; remove syringe.

   Figure 7

9. **Close skin**

   Suture wound.

   Suture cannula to skin.

   Figure 8

10. **Apply dressing**

    Apply povidone-iodine ointment to incision.

    Apply tincture of benzoin to skin.

    Apply sterile dressing.

    Securely tape dressing, *cannula,* and *stopcock.*

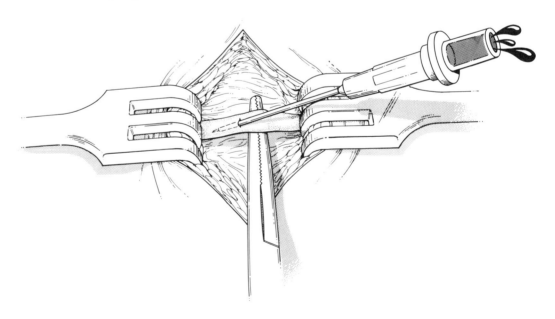

Figure 4
Cannulate artery.

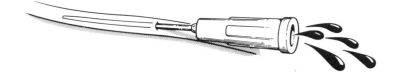

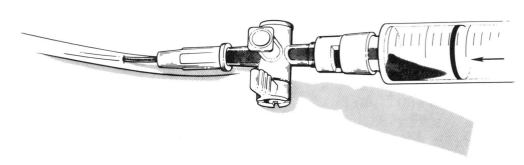

Figure 5
Advance cannula.

Figure 6
Flush cannula.

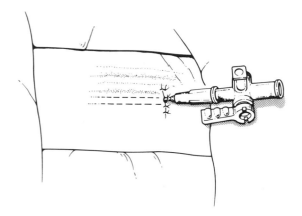

Figure 7
Close skin, suture cannula.

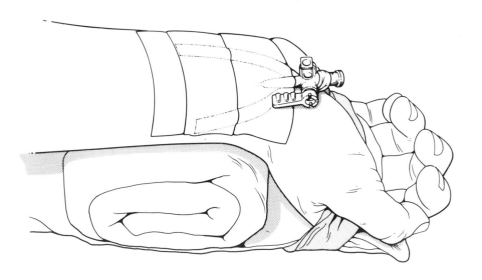

Figure 8
Apply dressing.

11. Attach transducer tubing

Securely tape or clip all connections.

12. Reapply armboard

Release tape on palm.

Remove towel.

Retape hand to armboard.

COMPLICATIONS

Same as with percutaneous procedure, Chapter 9.

SELECTED BIBLIOGRAPHY

1. Allen, E. V. Thromboangiitis obliterans; methods of diagnosis of chronic occlusive arterial lesions distal to the wrist with illustrative cases. *Am. J. Med. Sci.* 178:237, 1929.

    Description by Allen of the Allen test.

2. Barr, P. Percutaneous puncture of the radial artery with a multi-purpose Teflon catheter for indwelling use. *Acta Physiol. Scand.* 51:343, 1961.

    One of the first reports of arterial cannulation using the method described by Massa.

3. Evans, D., and Ozer, S. A simple method of arterial cannulation. *Can. Anaesth. Soc. J.* 17:181, 1970.

    Description of the transfixion technique.

4. Foti, P. R., and Moser, K. M. An effective, simple technique for indwelling arterial cannulation with Teflon. *Angiology* 20:439, 1969.

    Description of needle/cannula/stylette combination (Becton-Dickson) used with the transfixion technique.

5. Lowenstein, E., Little, J. W., III, and Lo, H. H. Prevention of cerebral embolization from flushing radial-artery cannulas. *N. Engl. J. Med.* 285:1414, 1971.

    Studies showing that injection in radial artery of boluses as small as 3 ml (average, 7 ml) were sufficient to cause cerebral embolization via retrograde flow in the arm.

6. Massa, D. J., Lundy, J. S., Faulconer, A., Jr., et al. A plastic needle. *Mayo Clin. Proc.* 25:413, 1950.

    One of the first reports of the needle in a cannula technique but used for venous cannulation.

7. Mortensen, J. D. Clinical sequelae from arterial needle puncture, cannulation and incision. *Circulation* 35:1118, 1967.

    A catalog of the many complications seen, especially with brachial artery puncture (when done for arteriography).

11.
Pulmonary Artery Catheterization with Balloon Flotation (Swan-Ganz) Catheter

Method of Garry F. Fitzpatrick

INDICATIONS

Measurement of pulmonary artery pressure

Indirect measurement of left atrial pressure

Measurement of cardiac output

EQUIPMENT (see Appendix for sample kit)

Intravenous conduit

Established

Skin prep

Sterile sponges

Alcohol-acetone solution

Povidone-iodine solution

Sterile field

Towels, 4

Half sheet

Towel clips

Local anesthesia

Syringe, 5-ml

Needles

25-gauge × ⅝-inch

21-gauge × 1½-inch

Lidocaine 1%, 10 ml

Venous access

   Cutdown set

   or

   Subclavian set with Angiocath or other over-the-needle cannula, #16

      Introducer: Cook or Desilet-Hoffman introducer of appropriate size for balloon catheter

   Scalpel blade, #11

Figure 1

Catheter insertion

   Balloon flotation (Swan-Ganz) catheters

      Double-lumen catheter, #5 Fr. or #7 Fr.

      or

      Triple-lumen catheter, #7 Fr. (for CVP and PA pressures)

      or

      Quadruple-lumen thermodilution "cardiac output" catheter, #7 Fr.

   Monitoring system

      Strain-gauge pressure transducer, connecting tubing, and 3-way stopcocks

      ECG monitor (oscilloscope preferred)

      Pressure recorder (sensitivity 1 cm deflection per 5 mm Hg)

      Portable x-ray or fluoroscope

      Heparinized saline (1000 units/100 ml)

   Syringe

      10-ml

      1-ml tuberculin

   Suture, 3-0 silk

   Needle holder

   Suture scissors

Dressing

   Sterile sponges

   Povidone-iodine ointment

   Adhesive tape, 1-inch

Catheter maintenance

   Heparin-saline constant infusion

Emergency equipment

   Defibrillator

Balloon tip

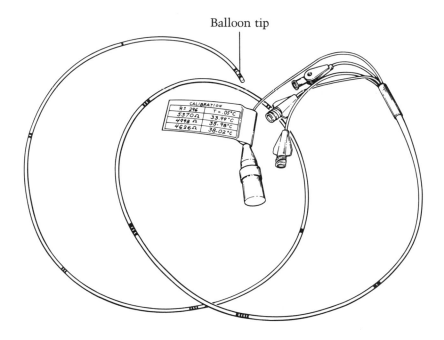

Figure 1
Pulmonary artery balloon
flotation (Swan-Ganz)
catheter (quadruple lumen
thermodilution type).

POSITION

Supine

Internal jugular approach: 10–20 degrees Trendelenburg

Antecubital fossa approach: Arm abducted 90 degrees

TECHNIQUE

1. Prep and drape

2. Use mask, gown, and gloves

3. Infiltrate local anesthetic

4. Test catheter balloon for leaks

   Inject air with balloon underwater.

5. Insert catheter in vein

Figure 2

   Use cutdown technique, Chapter 2, antecubital vein.

   or

   Insert into right internal jugular vein, percutaneously, as in internal jugular cannulation, Chapter 4, but use #16 Angiocath.

   Cannulate vein with #16 Angiocath.

Figure 3A

   Slide guide wire through Angiocath.

Figure 3B

   Remove Angiocath; replace with introducer and sleeve (nick skin first with #11 blade), and remove guide wire.

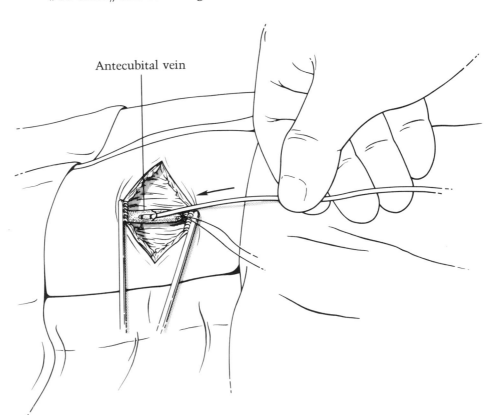

Antecubital vein

Figure 2
Catheter insertion via peripheral vein cutdown.

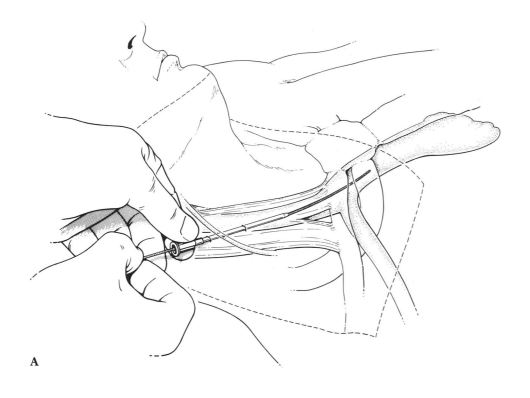

A

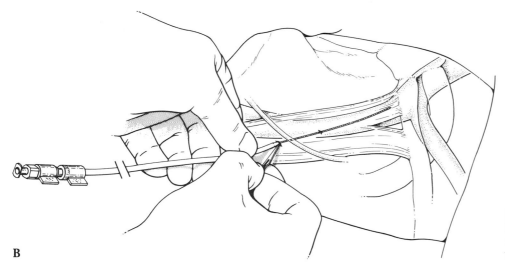

B

Figure 3A, B
Percutaneous catheter in-
sertion via internal jugular
vein.

Figure 3C   Remove introducer; leave sleeve in place.

Occlude end with finger to prevent air embolism or excessive bleeding.

Figure 3D   Slide PA catheter through introducer sleeve.

Return table to level position.

6. Advance catheter centrally

From right antecubital fossa	35–40 cm
From left antecubital fossa	45–50 cm
From internal jugular vein	10–15 cm
From subclavian vein	10 cm
From femoral vein	35–45 cm

The *left* antecubital fossa more regularly gains successful entry to the pulmonary artery than does the *right* antecubital fossa, as there is only a unidirectional arc in the catheter: $\mathcal{G}$ vs. $\mathcal{U}$.

7. Monitor pressure through PA lumen

Attach 3-way stopcock to PA lumen.

Flush with heparinized saline periodically through stopcock sidearm.

Connect other arm of stopcock to pressure monitor.

Respiratory fluctuations indicate intrathoracic position.

Calibrate recorder with strain gauge 5 cm below angle of Louis.

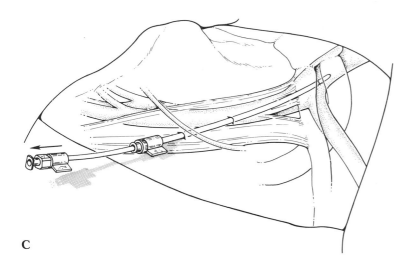

C

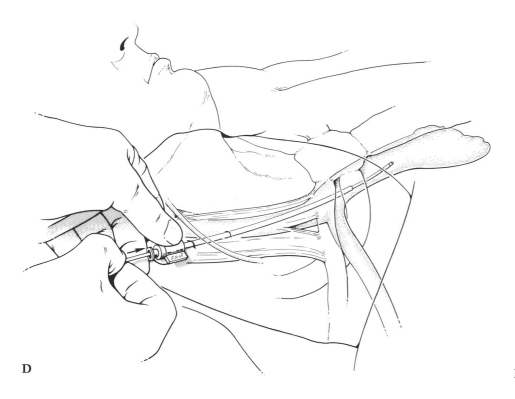

D

Figure 3C, D

8. Advance catheter through right heart

Inflate balloon, no more than recommended volume.

> (Because of danger of air embolism in patients with right-to-left shunt, use carbon dioxide rather than air.)

Observe pressure tracing *and* ECG: Deflate balloon and pull catheter back if multiple PVCs are elicited.

Figures 4, 5

Advance catheter into pulmonary artery until occluded pulmonary artery pressure (PA occl.) is obtained.

Fluoroscopy facilitates passage of catheter.

9. Confirm proper position in proximal pulmonary artery

Criteria

PA occl. (or wedge) pressure lower than PA pressure and returns to PA pressure promptly and consistently with balloon deflation

Characteristic PA and PA occl. pressure waves obtainable

No rise in PA occl. pressure on flushing catheter

Fully saturated (pulmonary venous) blood obtainable from occluded segment

X-ray confirms tip in right or left pulmonary artery

10. Secure catheter

Close cutdown incision if present.

Slide introducer sleeve (if present) out of vein.

Suture catheter to skin at point of entry.

11. Initiate constant heparin-saline flush

Concentration: 1000 units heparin/100 ml 0.9% saline

Rate: 2–3 ml/hour

12. Apply dressing

Apply povidone-iodine ointment.

Apply sterile sponge.

Tape securely.

13. Obtain portable chest x-ray

Rule out pneumothorax or hemothorax.

Confirm proper catheter position.

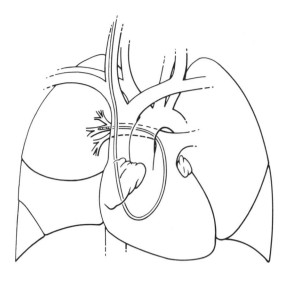

Figure 4
Advance catheter through right heart.

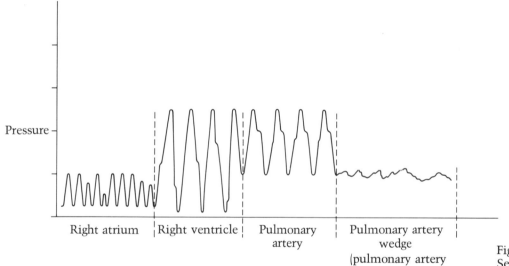

Pressure

Right atrium | Right ventricle | Pulmonary artery | Pulmonary artery wedge (pulmonary artery occluded)

Figure 5
Sequential pressure tracings.

CARE OF CATHETER

Adjust catheter position as necessary

As catheter softens at body temperature, transcardiac loop may shorten and allow distal catheter migration.

Result

PA pressure no longer obtainable; persistent PA occl. (or wedge) pressure present.

or

Only small volume necessary to obtain PA occl. pressure.

May cause local pulmonary infarction.

Withdraw catheter 1–2 cm if above occurs.

Continue constant infusion

Do not leave balloon inflated

Obtain daily chest x-ray

Look for pulmonary infarction or catheter migration.

Change dressing 3 times per week

Use technique of subclavian vein cannulation described in Chapter 3.

COMPLICATIONS

Arrhythmias

Etiology

Irritation of right heart by catheter tip during insertion; catheter "recoil" from PA back into sensitive right ventricular outflow tract.

Prevention

Always have balloon inflated when advancing catheter.

Have defibrillator immediately available.

Have intravenous infusion running for rapid administration of drugs as needed.

Withdraw catheter from right ventricle if multiple PVCs occur.

Pulmonary infarction

Etiology

Balloon left inflated.

Persistent undetected wedging of the catheter tip.

Prevention

Withdraw catheter slightly in case of distal catheter migration; check position of catheter by x-ray daily; monitor catheter tip pressure every 30 minutes.

Never leave balloon inflated for more than 1–2 minutes.

Monitor pulmonary capillary wedge pressure only intermittently.

If PA pressure damped, flush catheter.

If still damped, withdraw catheter 1–2 cm.

Rupture of pulmonary artery

Etiology

Overinflation of balloon in distal small vessel.

Prevention

Do not use fluid as inflation medium.

Never inflate balloon beyond recommended amount.

If resistance encountered, stop inflating and check catheter position by x-ray.

Perforation of pulmonary artery

Etiology

Advancement of catheter with balloon uninflated.

Catheter "migration."

Prevention

Advance catheter only with balloon inflated.

Correct catheter migration promptly.

Cardiac tamponade

Etiology

Perforation of right ventricle by catheter tip.

Prevention

Advance catheter only with balloon inflated.

Thromboembolism

Etiology

Clot formation on catheter.

Prevention

Sometimes unavoidable, often unpredictable, difficult to diagnose.

In hypercoagulable states, consider anticoagulation while catheter is in place.

If thrombosis or embolism is suspected or documented, remove catheter.

Septic phlebitis

Etiology

Infection, usually originating at the catheter insertion site.

Prevention

Adhere strictly to central venous line dressing protocol (see Chapter 3).

Suture catheter to skin to prevent movement of catheter in and out at skin insertion site.

Traumatic endocarditis

Etiology

Catheter trauma to tricuspid and pulmonary valves and right ventricular myocardium leading to vegetations and thromboembolization.

Prevention

Remove catheter as soon as possible.

Balloon rupture

Etiology

Overinflation of balloon.

Repeated gas sterilization and reuse of catheters.

Prevention

Avoid overinflation.

Restrict balloon flotation catheters to a single use.

Catheter kinking or knotting

Etiology

Insertion of excessive length of catheter or advancement of catheter too rapidly.

Prevention

Avoid advancing catheter greatly beyond distance at which entrance to ventricle is anticipated, especially if fluoroscopy unavailable.

Electrical hazards

Etiology

Catheter fluid column provides low impedance pathway to central circulation; danger of inducing serious cardiac dysrhythmias always present.

Prevention

Isolate and ground all electrical devices associated with intracardiac catheters.

Complications of subclavian and internal jugular cannulation

See Chapters 3 and 4.

SELECTED BIBLIOGRAPHY

1. Anderson, W. P., Dunegan, J. F., Knight, D. C., et al. Rapid estimation of pulmonary extravascular water with an instream catheter. *J. Appl. Physiol.* 39:843, 1975.

   Innovative future uses of flow-directed heart catheters in man. Brief report of experiment conducted in an animal model.

2. Fitzpatrick, G. F., Hampson, L. G., and Burgess, J. H. Bedside determination of left atrial pressure. *J. Can. Med. Assoc.* 106:1293, 1972.

   First demonstration in man that "balloon-occluded" pulmonary artery pressures are an accurate reflection of mean left atrial pressure.

3. Foote, G. A., Schabel, S. I., and Hodges, M. Pulmonary complications of the flow-directed balloon-tipped catheter. *N. Engl. J. Med.* 290:927, 1974.

   First large series that critically reviewed the hazards of flow-directed catheters and documented the incidence of complications associated with their use.

4. Swan, H. J. C., and Ganz, W. Use of balloon flotation catheters in critically ill patients. *Surg. Clin. N. Am.* 55:501, 1975.

   Summarizes 5 years' experience and states the clinical indications and uses of the Swan-Ganz catheter in critically ill patients.

5. Swan, H. J. C., Ganz, W., Forrester, J., et al. Catheterization of the heart in man with use of a flow-directed balloon-tipped catheter. *N. Engl. J. Med.* 283:447, 1970.

   Classic paper which first demonstrated the method and clinical usefulness of flow-directed flotation catheters at the bedside.

12.
Temporary Transvenous Pacemaker Placement

Method of John A. Paraskos

INDICATIONS

Symptomatic bradycardia from

Complete heart block

High degree second degree heart block

Sinus bradycardia

Threatened complete heart block

Anterior myocardial infarction with new bundle branch block

Stokes-Adams attacks with trifascicular block

Preoperatively in selected patients

Ventricular irritability in selected cases

Ventricular asystole

Caution: During cardiac arrest cardiopulmonary resuscitation takes precedence over pacing. With life-threatening bradycardia, infuse epinephrine or isoproterenol to accelerate an idioventricular pacemaker while transvenous catheter positioned.

EQUIPMENT (see Appendix for sample kit)

Monitoring

ECG machine

Skin prep

Alcohol-acetone solution

Povidone-iodine solution

Sterile sponges

Sterile field

   Mask, gown, gloves

   Towels, 4

   Towel clips

   Half sheet

Local anesthetic

   Syringe, 5-ml

   Needles

      25-gauge × ⅝-inch

      22-gauge × 1½-inch

   Lidocaine 1%, 10 ml

Figure 1   Catheter insertion

   Pacing catheter, lightweight, semifloating, bipolar (we prefer Elecath catheter with introducing cannula supplied in kit)

   Skin suture, 3-0

   Suture scissors

Dressing

   Povidone-iodine ointment

   Sterile sponges

   Tincture of benzoin

   Adhesive tape, 2-inch

POSITION

Supine

10–20-degrees Trendelenburg

Head turned to opposite side

Roll under shoulders

TECHNIQUE

1. **Monitor ECG continuously**

2. **Prep and drape neck**

3. **Use mask, gown, and gloves**

Figure 2   4. **Cannulate vein**

Use Elecath introducing cannula (over-the-needle cannula supplied with kit).

Use either subclavian (Chapter 3) or internal jugular vein (Chapter 4) cannulation.

Note: Use of antecubital veins for insertion causes increased incidence of catheter motion and dislodgment.

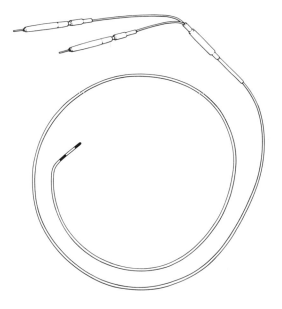

Figure 1
Pacing catheter.

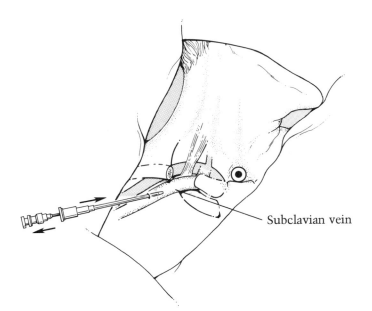

Subclavian vein

Figure 2
Cannulate vein.

Figure 3

5. Insert electrode catheter

Place gentle 45-degree curve in distal 5 cm of electrode catheter.

Slide through introducing cannula.

Withdraw cannula over electrode catheter.

Return bed to level position.

6. Fluoroscopic positioning of electrode (preferred method)

Slide electrode catheter through superior vena cava (SVC) into right atrium (RA).

Figure 4A

Position catheter tip against lateral wall of RA.

Twist catheter until distal end is seen twisting.

Simultaneously advance catheter across tricuspid valve, through right ventricle (RV), and into pulmonary artery to confirm proper passage through RV.

Slowly withdraw electrode until in RV.

Advance tip to RV apex.

Figure 4B

Wedge catheter gently into trabeculae—catheter tip near left heart border on PA x-ray and near anterior heart border on lateral x-ray.

Figure 4C

Withdraw catheter to remove any redundancy—catheter should lie in smooth arc from SVC to RV.

Ascertain electrode stability fluoroscopically—wide swings of catheter tip during systole, respiration, and body movement indicate improper position.

Frequent ventricular premature beats, or ventricular tachycardia or fibrillation, demand immediate withdrawal of electrode into SVC (until irritability ceases and/or is appropriately treated). Then reposition.

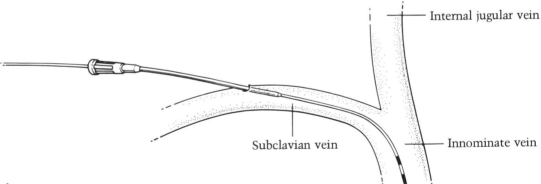

Figure 3
Insert electrode catheter.

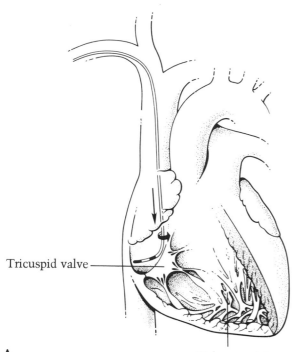

Tricuspid valve

A

Right ventricle

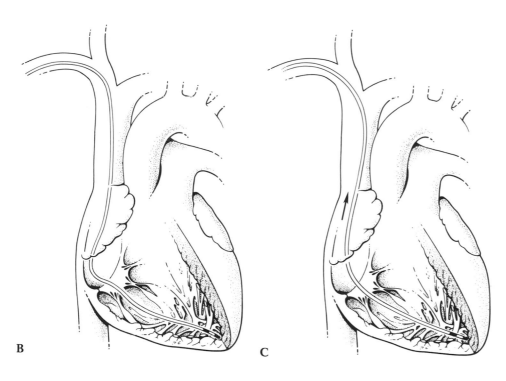

B

C

Figure 4
Fluoroscopic positioning
of electrode.

6A. Electrocardiographic positioning of electrode

(Used in emergency situations when fluoroscopy is unavailable and patient has spontaneous ventricular electrical activity)

Slide electrode catheter into SVC.

Attach precordial electrode from ECG to external end of distal electrode. Attach limb leads in standard fashion.

Record on V lead.

Advance catheter into right ventricle and position.

ECG pattern localizes electrode tip.

Figure 5

6B. "Blind" or "turned-on" positioning of electrode

(Used in emergency situations, particularly when no intrinsic electrical activity exists)

Slide electrode catheter into SVC.

Attach external end to pacemaker generator.

Turn generator on: rate ~70/min; highest output.

Advance catheter until ventricular pacing occurs.

Confirm position radiographically as soon as possible.

7. Establish pacing

Pacing generator setting

Off

Demand mode

Output

0 milliamperes

Rate

Physiological range (~70) but faster than patient's rate

Connect external end of electrode to external pacing generator.

Bipolar electrode

Distal end to negative terminal, proximal end to positive terminal

Unipolar electrode

Subcutaneous needle to positive terminal, electrode to negative terminal

(Avoid placing needle in muscle or in contact with pacing catheter.)

Turn generator to "on."

Slowly increase output until ECG documents ventricular pacing: pacing spike followed immediately by wide QRS

Perform 12 lead ECG and document left bundle branch block pattern. If right bundle branch block pattern exists, electrode position is incorrect.

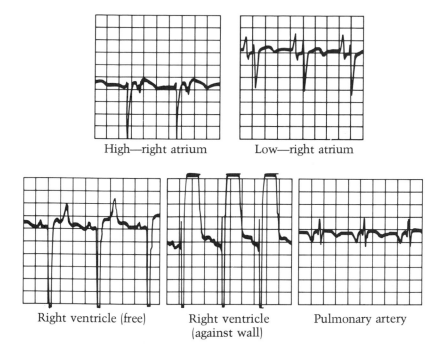

High—right atrium   Low—right atrium

Right ventricle (free)   Right ventricle (against wall)   Pulmonary artery

Figure 5
Electrocardiographic positioning of electrode.

8. **Establish pacing threshold**

   Slowly decrease generator output.

   Threshold

   Output at which pacing ceases (should be 1 mA or less)

9. **Resume pacing at output 2 mA above threshold**

10. **Secure catheter**

    Suture catheter at skin entrance point.

11. **Apply dressing**

    Apply povidone-iodine ointment to skin puncture site.

    Form two small loops of sterile catheter adjacent to puncture site.

    Apply 4-inch × 4-inch sponge, incorporating loops.

    Apply tincture of benzoin to skin.

    Tape securely.

12. **Obtain PA and lateral chest film to confirm proper position**

COMPLICATIONS

Myocardial perforation

Etiology

   Excessive advancement of stiff electrode into RV apex.

Prevention

   Advance catheter gently.

   Avoid using stiff catheters.

   (No therapy usually required other than to withdraw catheter. Bleeding or tamponade unusual.)

Catheter displacement

Etiology

   Poor initial electrode placement.

   Excessive redundancy in catheter course.

   Inadequate anchoring.

Prevention

   Withdraw redundant catheter carefully.

Figure 4C

   Observe correct catheter tip "entrapment" in apex of RV.

   Carefully suture in place.

Diaphragmatic pacing

Etiology

Catheter displacement into RA and pacing of phrenic nerve; or myocardial perforation with direct diaphragmatic pacing.

Prevention

As for myocardial perforation and catheter displacement.

Increased ventricular irritability

Etiology

Impingement of catheter on a "sensitive" area of ventricular endocardium.

Prevention

Reposition catheter.

Increased threshold to pacing or loss of pacing

Etiology

Catheter displacement, myocardial perforation, generator failure (battery failure), poor contact of electrode pins to generator, frayed or broken electrode wire, inflammation of myocardium at catheter tip, or necrosis or scarring of RV apex.

Prevention

Reposition catheter, replace electrode as indicated.

SELECTED BIBLIOGRAPHY

1. Atkins, J. M., Leshin, S. J., Blomqvist, G., et al.   Ventricular conduction blocks and sudden death in acute myocardial infarction. Potential indications for pacing. *N. Engl. J. Med.* 288:281, 1973.

   Discusses specific indications for patients with acute myocardial infarction.

2. Castellanos, A., Jr., Zuckerman, W., and Berkovits, B. V.   Cardiac Pacemakers. In D. E. Harken (ed.), *Cardiac Surgery 2.* Philadelphia: Davis, 1971.

   Discusses indications for pacing.

3. Chardack, W.M.   Cardiac Pacemakers and Heart Block. In D. C. Sabiston, Jr. et al. (eds.), *Gibbon's Surgery of the Chest* (3d ed.). Philadelphia: Saunders, 1976.

   Good review including more recent developments.

4. Furman, S.   Fundamentals of cardiac pacing. *Am. Heart J.* 73:261, 1967.

   Good review of basics including history, medications, and physiology.

5. Furman, S., and Escher, D. J. W.   *Principles and Techniques of Cardiac Pacing.* New York: Harper & Row, 1970.

   Review including description of procedure for insertion.

6. Lown, B., and Kosowsky, B. D.   Artificial cardiac pacemakers I, II, III. *N. Engl. J. Med.* 283:907, 971, 1023, 1970.

   Excellent review of history, medications, and "trouble-shooting."

7. Rubin, I., Arbeit, S. R., and Gross, H.   The electrocardiographic recognition of pacemaker function and failure. *Ann. Intern. Med.* 71:603, 1969.

   Description of ECG patterns of pacer failure.

13.
Pericardiocentesis

Method of Ira S. Ockene

INDICATIONS

Emergency relief of cardiac tamponade

Drainage of pericardial effusion

Removal of pericardial fluid to establish the etiology of a pericardial effusion

EQUIPMENT (see Appendix for sample kit)

Skin prep

Sterile sponges

Alcohol-acetone solution

Povidone-iodine solution

Sterile field

Mask, gown, gloves

Towels

Towel clips

Local anesthetic

Syringe, 10-ml

Needles

25-gauge × ⅝-inch

21-gauge × 1½-inch

Lidocaine 1%, 10 ml

Pericardiocentesis

Syringes

10-ml

50-ml

Stopcock, 3-way

Connecting tubing for stopcock

Needle-catheter (Subclavian Jugular Catheter kit with metal-hubbed, #14 needle [Deseret])

Needle, 2¾-inch, 18-gauge spinal

Alligator clip, sterile

ECG machine, electrically isolated

Collecting basin, sterile

Fluid analysis

Culture tubes

Hematocrit tubes

Cytology tubes

Dressing

Sterile sponges

Adhesive tape, 1-inch

Povidone-iodine ointment

TECHNIQUE

1. Attach ECG limb leads to patient

2. Use mask, gown, gloves

Figure 1   **3. Prep and drape**

Upper abdomen and lower chest

4. Infiltrate local anesthetic

Use lidocaine 1%.

Inject at left xiphocostal angle.

Infiltrate deep to costal arch.

Aspirate carefully after needle advancement—may demonstrate pericardial fluid.

Figure 2   **5. Insert pericardiocentesis needle**

Connect metal needle (from Subclavian Jugular Catheter kit) to V lead with sterile alligator clip, and place 10-ml syringe on needle.

Insert needle in anesthetized tract.

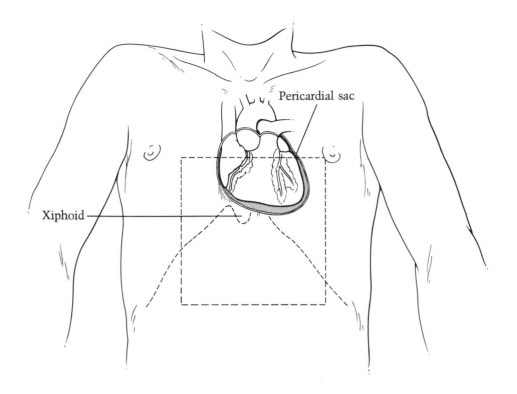

Figure 1
Prep and drape.

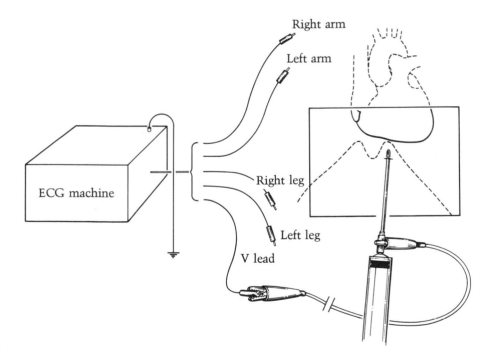

Figure 2
Insert pericardiocentesis
needle.

Figure 3

When needle tip is deep to costal arch, depress hub and advance needle toward left shoulder, aspirating during advancement.

Continually monitor V lead on ECG for injury current.

Figure 4

S-T segment elevation is present with ventricular epicardial contact.

P-R segment elevation is present with atrial epicardial contact.

A sudden "give" or "pop" may be felt with pericardial puncture.

Epicardial contact is felt through needle as grating sensation.

With epicardial contact, withdraw needle slightly, and reposition to obtain pericardial fluid.

If fluid not obtained, redirect needle toward head or right shoulder.

Figure 5

6. Remove pericardial fluid

Confirm intrapericardial position by fluid withdrawal.

Remove syringe.

Slide catheter through needle into pericardial space; slide needle off catheter; screw hub onto catheter.

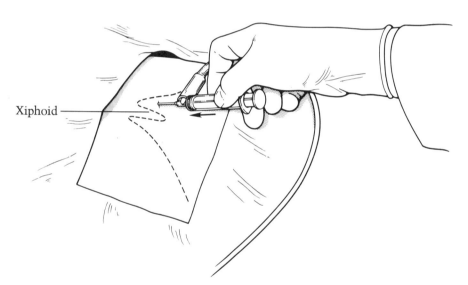

Figure 3
Advance and aspirate.

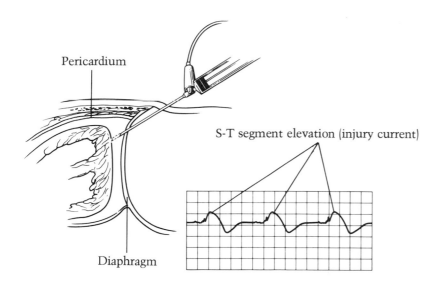

Pericardium

Diaphragm

S-T segment elevation (injury current)

Figure 4
Monitor V lead for injury current.

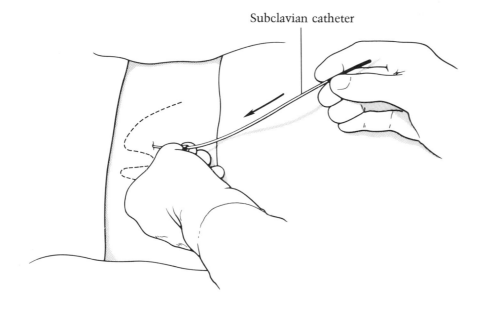

Subclavian catheter

Figure 5
Slide cannula into pericardial space through needle.

Figure 6

Attach 50-ml syringe and stopcock.

Withdraw fluid.

Ventricular puncture suggested if fluid bloody and clots or if hematocrit of fluid same as peripheral venous blood.

If doubt exists as to catheter location, inject Decholin (sodium dehydrocholate), 3 ml. If patient tastes bitter substance, myocardial puncture is present—remove catheter.

Send fluid for studies as indicated

Cell count

Protein

Cytology

Culture

Gram stain

If catheter left in for drainage, apply povidone-iodine ointment, sterile dressing, and tape.

7. Withdraw catheter

8. Apply dressing

Sterile gauze and adhesive tape

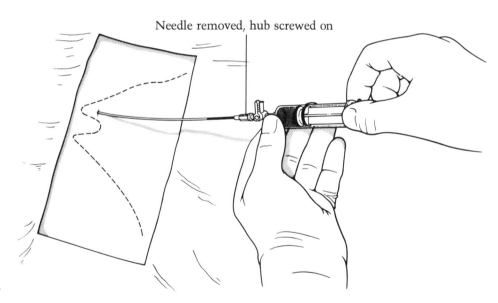
Needle removed, hub screwed on

Figure 6
Withdraw pericardial fluid.

ALTERNATIVE PROCEDURE—FOR DIAGNOSTIC PERICARDIOCENTESIS ONLY

1–4. Same as in general technique

5. Insert pericardiocentesis needle

Connect metal needle hub (from 2¾-inch 18-gauge spinal needle) to V lead with sterile alligator clip and place 50-ml syringe on needle.

Insert needle in anesthetized tract.

When needle tip is deep to costal arch, depress hub and advance needle toward left shoulder, aspirating during advancement.

Continually monitor V lead on ECG for injury current.

S-T segment elevation is present with ventricular epicardial contact.

P-R segment elevation is present with atrial epicardial contact.

A sudden "give" or "pop" may be felt with pericardial puncture.

Epicardial contact is felt through needle as grating sensation.

With epicardial contact, withdraw needle slightly and reposition to obtain pericardial fluid.

If fluid not obtained, redirect needle toward head or right shoulder.

6. Remove pericardial fluid

Confirm intrapericardial position by fluid withdrawal.

Ventricular puncture suggested if fluid bloody and clots or if hematocrit of fluid same as peripheral venous blood.

If doubt exists as to catheter location, inject Decholin (sodium dehydrocholate), 3 ml. If patient tastes bitter substance, myocardial puncture present—remove needle.

Send fluid for studies as indicated

Cell count

Protein

Cytology

Culture

Gram stain

7. Withdraw needle

8. Apply dressing

Sterile gauze and adhesive tape

COMPLICATIONS

Ventricular puncture

Etiology

Advancement of needle into ventricular cavity.

Prevention

Monitor for injury current on ECG.

Advance needle slowly, rotating hub and aspirating.

Therapy

Withdraw needle until blood is no longer obtained and/or S-T changes disappear.

Most ventricular punctures have no sequelae; monitor patient and observe for tamponade.

Arrhythmias

Etiology

Irritation of ventricular or atrial myocardium by needle.

Prevention

Withdraw needle when arrhythmias or S-T segment deviation occurs.

Use electrically isolated ECG machine; older machines can carry a significant shock hazard and may *cause* ventricular arrhythmias, including ventricular fibrillation.

SELECTED BIBLIOGRAPHY

1. Bishop, L. H., Jr., Estes, E. H., Jr., and McIntosh, H. D.   The electrocardiogram as a safeguard in pericardiocentesis. *J.A.M.A.* 162:264, 1956.

   Original discussion of electrocardiographic monitoring of pericardiocentesis.

2. Fredriksen, R. T., Cohen, L. S., and Mullins, C. B.   Pericardial windows or pericardiocentesis for pericardial effusions. *Am. Heart J.* 82:158, 1971.

   Good discussion of the merits of pericardiocentesis vs. open drainage.

3. Kilpatrick, Z. M., and Chapman, C. B.   On pericardiocentesis. *Am. J. Cardiol.* 16:722, 1965.

   Excellent historical review.

4. Neill, J. R., Hurst, J. W., and Penfold, E. L. J.   A pericardiocentesis electrode. *N. Engl. J. Med.* 264:711, 1961.

   More sophisticated approach to electrocardiographic monitoring during pericardiocentesis.

5. Schaffer, A. I.   Pericardiocentesis with the aid of a plastic catheter and ECG monitor. *Am. J. Cardiol.* 4:83, 1959.

   Description of the procedure modified by using a flexible plastic cannula.

6. Spodick, D. H.   Acute cardiac tamponade: Pathologic physiology, diagnosis and management. *Prog. Cardiovasc. Dis.* 10:64, 1967.

   Comprehensive review of cardiac tamponade including the role of pericardiocentesis.

14.
Defibrillation and Emergency Cardioversion

Method of
John P. Howe III

INDICATIONS

Life-threatening ventricular or atrial arrhythmias

Indications for defibrillation

Ventricular fibrillation

In ventricular fibrillation due to inadequate ventilation, adequate ventilation must precede defibrillation.

Indications for cardioversion

Ventricular tachycardia, unresponsive to lidocaine

Atrial fibrillation, flutter, or other ectopic atrial tachycardia complicated by hypotension or severe left heart failure

Contraindications for cardioversion

Digitalis intoxication in supraventricular tachycardia

Figure 1

EQUIPMENT (see Appendix for sample kit)

Defibrillation or cardioversion

Direct current cardioverter with

Oscilloscopic monitor

Selection switches for energy level and storage

Synchronization mode

Electrode paddles (usually 9-cm diameter)

Electrode jelly or saline gauze 4-inch × 4-inch pads

Note: Do not use alcohol pads (flammable).

Sedation

(Amnesic drug for awake patients only)

Diazepam (Valium) 10 mg/ampule

or

Thiopental sodium (Pentothal) 500 mg/vial

or

Methohexital sodium (Brevital) 500 mg/vial

(Sterile water required to mix with Pentothal and Brevital)

Resuscitation

Oxygen with bag-valve-mask device

Venous access

Intravenous cannula (plastic), IV tubing, 5% dextrose

Emergency drugs

Lidocaine, 2%

Procainamide, 100 mg/ml

Atropine, 0.4 mg/ml

Isoproterenol, 0.2 mg/ml

POSITION

Supine

Firm underlying surface

TECHNIQUE: DEFIBRILLATION

1. **Turn cardioverter** *on*

2. **Turn synchronizer switch** *off*

3. **Select energy level at highest output (usually 300–400 watt-seconds)**

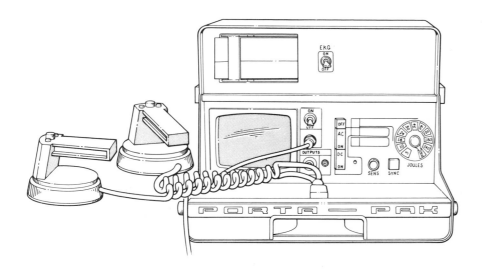

Figure 1
Defibrillation or cardioversion equipment.

Figure 2

4. **Reduce skin resistance**

   Apply electrode jelly to paddles

   or

   Apply saline pads to skin at appropriate position.

   Note: Do not use alcohol pads, which might ignite.

5. **Apply paddles**

   Paddle #1: below right clavicle just lateral to upper sternum

   Paddle #2: just lateral to left nipple in anterior axillary line

6. **Assure no patient or bed contact by operator or assistants**

7. **Administer shock**

8. **Check pulse, electrocardiogram, and airway**

9. **If unsuccessful, continue cardiopulmonary resuscitation (including appropriate drugs) and then repeat defibrillation**

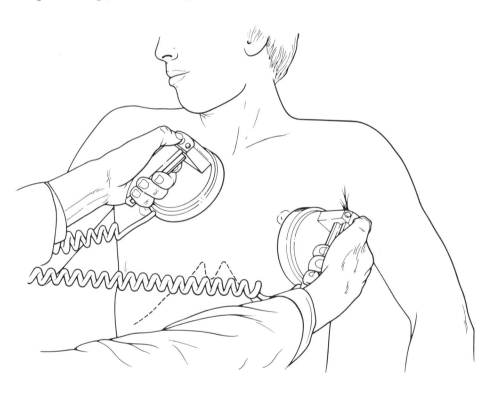

Figure 2
Apply paddles.

COMPLICATIONS: DEFIBRILLATION

Absence of defibrillator current

Etiology

Defibrillator not charged.

Synchronizer switch on.

Prevention

Plug defibrillator into electrical outlet switch.

Switch synchronizer off.

Skin burns

Etiology

Inadequate electrode contact with skin, causing sparking between paddle and skin.

Arcing between paddles.

Prevention

Layer electrode jelly or saline pads evenly between skin and paddles.

Apply paddles firmly to chest.

Prevent jelly or saline contact between paddle sites.

Electrical shock to operator or assistants

Etiology

Grounding of current through person touching patient or bed.

Prevention

Have all personnel stand back from bed before administering shock.

Assure no operator contact with jelly or saline on paddles.

TECHNIQUE: EMERGENCY CARDIOVERSION

1. **Attach patient electrodes to input mode of cardioverter**

2. **Turn cardioverter on**

3. **Turn synchronizer switch on**

   Ascertain that synchronizing signal falls on R wave.

4. **Select appropriate energy level**

   Ventricular tachycardia—200 watt-seconds

   Atrial arrhythmias—50 watt-seconds

5. **Give amnesic drug if patient awake**

6. **Reduce skin resistance**

   Apply electrode jelly to paddles

   or

   Apply saline pads to skin at appropriate position.

   Note: Do not use alcohol pads, which might ignite.

Figure 3

7. **Apply paddles (as in defibrillation)**

   Paddle #1: below right clavicle just lateral to upper sternum

   Paddle #2: just lateral to left nipple in anterior axillary line

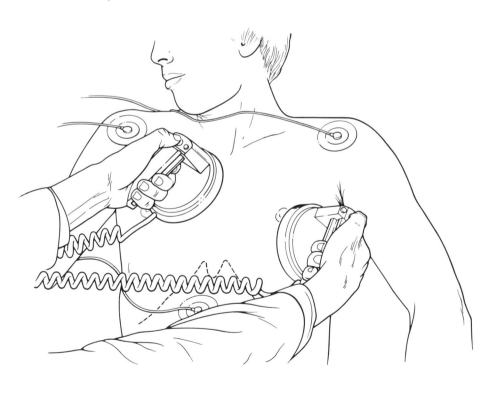

Figure 3
Apply paddles (as in
defibrillation).

8. **Assure no patient or bed contact by operator or assistant**

9. **Administer shock**

   Hold firing buttons down until patient receives current (as noted by muscle twitch).

10. **Check pulse, electrocardiogram, and airway**

11. **If rhythm does not revert, increase energy level and repeat cardioversion**

COMPLICATIONS: EMERGENCY CARDIOVERSION

1–3. **Same as complications of defibrillation**

4. **Cardiac muscle damage**

   Etiology

   Direct damage from electrical current.

   Prevention

   Use large paddles (9 cm or greater).

5. **Ventricular fibrillation**

   Etiology

   Shock administered during vulnerable period (on T wave).

   Prevention

   Ascertain that cardioverter senses R waves properly and that synchronizer signal falls on R wave.

   Confirm that synchronizer switch is on.

   Treatment

   Reset energy storage to maximum output.

   Turn synchronizer switch off.

   Defibrillate.

6. **Pulmonary edema (after conversion from atrial fibrillation)**

   Etiology

   Left atrial paralysis.

   Prevention

   Avoid high energy level for atrial cardioversion.

7. **Peripheral embolization**

   Etiology

   Dislodgment of intracardiac thrombosis.

   Prevention

   Not possible for emergency cardioversion (anticoagulate for elective cardioversion).

SELECTED BIBLIOGRAPHY

1. Dorney, E. R. The Use of Cardioversion and Pacemakers in the Management of Arrhythmias. In J. W. Hurst et al. (eds.), *The Heart* (3d ed.). New York: McGraw-Hill, 1974. Pp. 558–562.

   General discussion of various methods of cardioversion with extensive bibliography.

2. Lown, B., Neuman, J., Amarasingham, R., et al. Comparison of alternating current with direct current electroshock across the closed chest. *Am. J. Cardiol.* 10:223, 1962.

   Original work advocating the use of DC shock for cardiac defibrillation.

3. Parker, M. R. Defibrillation and Synchronized Cardioversion. In *Advanced Cardiac Life Support.* Dallas: American Heart Association, 1975.

   Straightforward presentation of AHA standards for defibrillation and emergency cardioversion.

4. Resnekov, L. Theory and practice of electroversion of cardiac dysrhythmias. *Med. Clin. North Am.* 60:325, 1976.

   Excellent review of recent literature, emphasizing drug therapy and follow-up studies.

15.
Nasotracheal Suctioning

Method of Joel M. Seidman

INDICATIONS

Removing tracheobronchial secretions

Obtaining sputum specimen

EQUIPMENT (see Appendix for sample kit)

Suction catheter with finger-occluded suction vent, usually #14 Fr. in adults

Suction source

Sputum trap

Gloves

Sterile water

Specimen container

Water-soluble lubricant

Oxygen mask and oxygen source

POSITION

Figure 1

Sitting with pillow for head support preferred

If not possible, semisitting or supine

TECHNIQUE

1. **Preoxygenate patient**

2. **Use gloves**

Figure 2

3. **Insert tube into nose**

    Interpose sputum trap between catheter and suction source.

    Lubricate distal end of catheter.

    Use more patent nostril.

    Advance catheter horizontally along floor of nose until tube curves into hypopharynx.

Figure 3

4. **Advance into trachea**

    Instruct patient to assume "sniffing position" of head and neck.

    Advance only during

      Deep breath preceding cough.

      Deep voluntary or spontaneous inspiration.

    Keep suction vent open during advancement.

    If intubation difficult, place gauze sponge around tongue and pull tongue forward—serves to move epiglottis forward and helps uncover glottis.

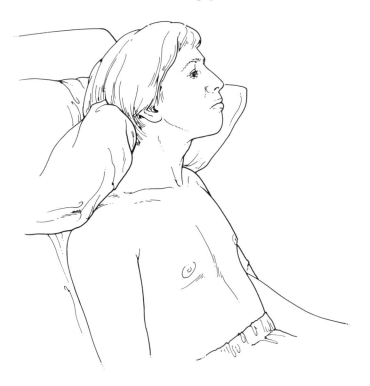

Figure 1
Position.

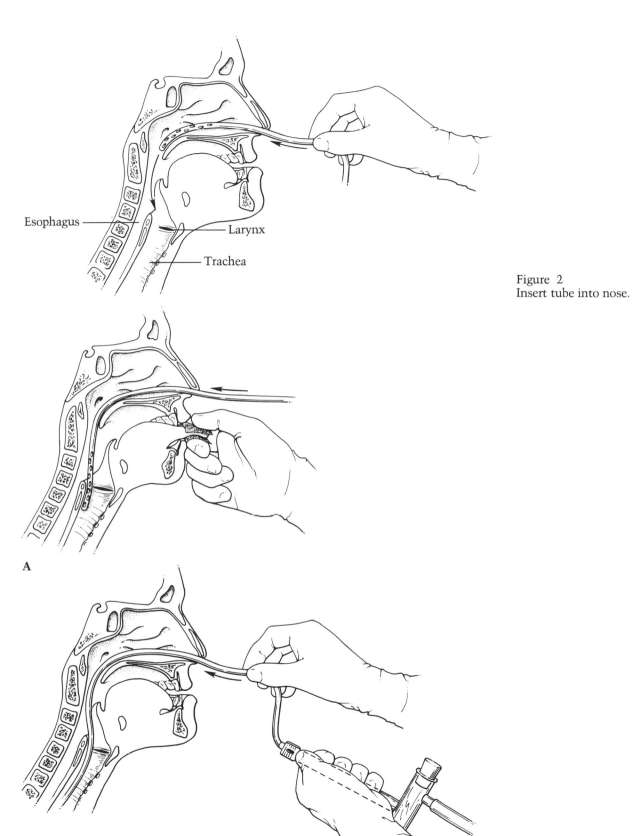

Esophagus

Larynx

Trachea

Figure 2
Insert tube into nose.

A

B

Figure 3
Advance into trachea.

5. Confirm intratracheal position

Passage into trachea usually causes coughing.

Tube through glottis always causes difficulty in phonation.

Figure 4

6. Apply suction

Intermittently occlude suction vent.

Maximum of 10 seconds at a time

7. Allow reoxygenation before resuctioning

Wait 30–60 seconds.

Avoid any suction on catheter during reoxygenation.

8. Remove catheter

COMPLICATIONS

Cardiac arrhythmia

Etiology

Vagal stimulation in presence of hypoxemia.

Prevention

Assure adequate oxygenation before and during procedure.

Avoid suctioning longer than 10 seconds without reoxygenation.

Bleeding

Etiology

Trauma to mucous membranes.

Prevention

Avoid forcing catheter.

A small amount of bleeding is common and is of no concern.

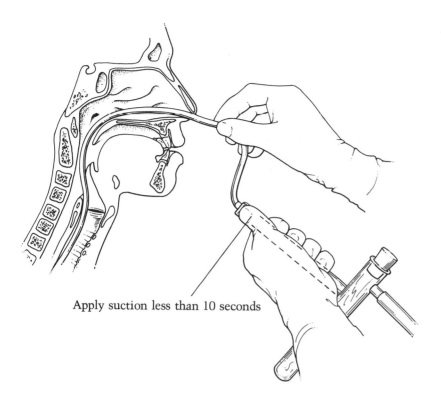

Apply suction less than 10 seconds

Figure 4
Apply suction.

SELECTED BIBLIOGRAPHY

1. Haight, C. Intratracheal suction in the management of postoperative pulmonary complications. *Ann. Surg.* 107:218, 1938.

   Early description of method and rationale.

2. Shim, C., Fine, N., Fernandez, R., et al. Cardiac arrhythmias resulting from tracheal suctioning. *Ann. Intern. Med.* 71:1149, 1969.

   Documentation of the prevention of cardiac arrhythmias during tracheal suctioning by prebreathing 100% oxygen instead of air.

16.
Transtracheal Aspiration (Cricothyroid Puncture)

Method of Joel M. Seidman

INDICATIONS

Diagnostic

Obtaining of sputum specimen uncontaminated by oropharyngeal organisms

When patient cannot raise sputum

When study of expectorated sputum is unrevealing or confusing

When patient is likely to be infected with unusual organism (immunosuppression, alcoholism, seizures, aspiration, lung abscess)

Therapeutic

Production of cough via tracheal stimulation in patients with poor cough

Caution: Not indicated in case of uncomplicated pulmonary infection with spontaneously expectorated sputum that gives adequate diagnostic information.

CONTRAINDICATIONS

Bleeding diathesis

Uncontrollable, severe cough

Uncooperative patient

Untreated hypoxemia

EQUIPMENT (see Appendix for sample kit)

Skin prep

Sterile sponges

Alcohol-acetone solution

Povidone-iodine solution

Sterile field

Fenestrated drape

Gloves

Local anesthetic

Syringe, 3-ml

Needle, 22-gauge × 1½-inch or 23-gauge × 1-inch

Lidocaine 1%, 5 ml, *without* epinephrine

Cannulation equipment

14-gauge (through-the-needle cannula) Intracath

Syringe, 10-ml

Nonbacteriostatic sterile saline

Culture media or transport containers

Routine

Anaerobic

Dressing

Band-Aid

Figure 1

POSITION

Supine

Pillow or roll under shoulders to extend neck

TECHNIQUE

Figure 2

1. Locate cricothyroid space

2. Use gloves

Figure 2

3. Prep and drape neck

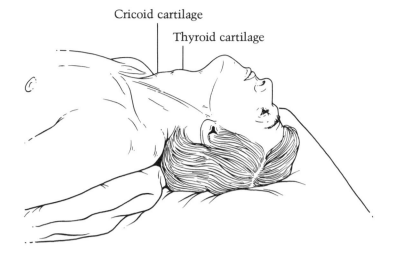

Cricoid cartilage

Thyroid cartilage

Figure 1
Position.

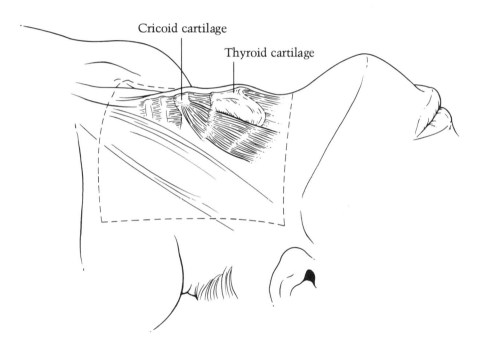

Cricoid cartilage

Thyroid cartilage

Figure 2
Locate cricothyroid space,
prep and drape neck.

Figure 3

4. Infiltrate local anesthetic

Raise skin wheal in midline over cricothyroid membrane.

Infiltrate down to membrane; avoid injecting lidocaine into trachea—it is bacteriostatic.

Figure 4

5. Puncture cricothyroid membrane

Use 14-gauge Intracath needle, bevel up, on syringe.

Aim caudad, 45 degrees to skin.

Hold needle 1.5 cm from point to avoid plunging too deeply.

Firmly thrust needle through membrane.

Aspirate to confirm intratracheal position.

Remove syringe.

Figure 5

Quickly thread catheter down into trachea.

If catheter does not thread easily, remove catheter and needle as unit; do *not* remove catheter separately. Then repeat cricothyroid puncture.

Remove stylette; slide needle out of trachea over cannula.

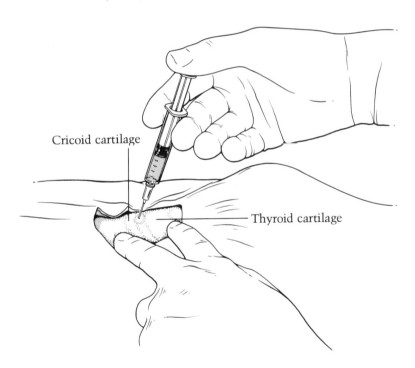

Figure 3
Infiltrate local anesthetic.

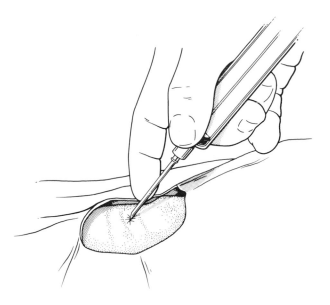

Figure 4
Puncture cricothyroid
membrane with Intracath
needle.

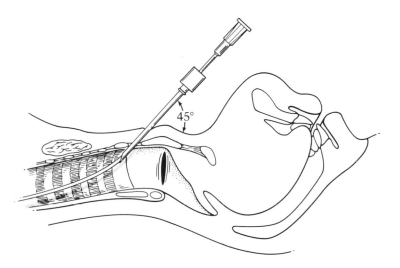

Figure 5
Thread catheter through
needle into trachea.

Figure 6

6. Aspirate specimen

Attach 10-ml syringe to cannula.

Aspirate during cough only.

Movement of intratracheal catheter will usually stimulate cough.

If specimen is inadequate or if spontaneous cough not present, inject 2–3 ml of sterile, nonbacteriostatic saline and aspirate again.

7. Remove syringe and inoculate media immediately

8. Withdraw catheter, apply dressing

Apply pressure for 5 minutes.

Apply Band-Aid.

9. Order bed rest for 8 hours

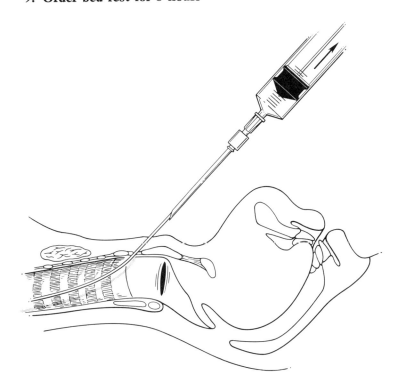

Figure 6
Aspirate specimen.

COMPLICATIONS

Bleeding into trachea

Etiology

Bleeding diathesis.

Entry into infracricoid venous plexus.

Prevention

Check bleeding studies if there is a history of bleeding diathesis.

Ensure puncture between thyroid and cricoid cartilages.

Note: A small amount of blood-tinged sputum is expected for several hours.

Treatment

Immediate endotracheal intubation indicated for hemoptysis that could compromise ventilation.

Subcutaneous or mediastinal emphysema

Etiology

Entry of air into subcutaneous tissue or mediastinum from trachea or skin surface.

Prevention

Do not perform in patient with uncontrollable or severe cough; apply pressure to puncture site for 5 minutes.

Prescribe bed rest for 8 hours after procedure.

Cardiac arrhythmia or arrest

Etiology

Vagal stimulation in hypoxemic patient.

Prevention

Ensure adequate oxygenation.

Catheter aspiration

Etiology

Catheter pulled back through needle, shearing off catheter at needle tip.

Prevention

When needle in trachea, never withdraw catheter through needle.

SELECTED BIBLIOGRAPHY

1. Bartlett, J. G., Rosenblatt, J. E., and Feingold, S. M.   Percutaneous transtracheal aspiration in the diagnosis of anaerobic pulmonary infection. *Ann. Intern. Med.* 79:535, 1973.

   Demonstrates success in isolation of anaerobes by transtracheal aspiration.

2. Kalinske, R. W., Parker, R. H., Brandt, D., et al.   Diagnostic usefulness and safety of transtracheal aspiration. *N. Engl. J. Med.* 276:604, 1967.

   Describes method of transtracheal aspiration and complication of subcutaneous or mediastinal emphysema. Demonstrates the frequency of contamination of expectorated sputum as compared with transtracheal aspirate.

3. Pecora, D. V.   A method of securing uncontaminated tracheal secretions for bacterial examination. *J. Thorac. Cardiovasc. Surg.* 37:653, 1959.

   Original description of method of transtracheal aspiration.

4. Spencer, C. D., and Beaty, H. N.   Complications of transtracheal aspiration. *N. Engl. J. Med.* 286:304, 1972.

   Case reports of three complications: bradycardia in hypoxemia, fatal hemorrhage with aspiration, and vomiting with aspiration.

17.
Endotracheal Intubation

Method of Adrian S. Selwyn

INDICATIONS

Airway maintenance

During general anesthesia

In emergency situations

Cardiac arrest

Respiratory failure

Severe upper airway obstruction (upper airway trauma may preclude endotracheal intubation and require emergency cricothyroidotomy)

Head and neck injuries

Severe facial burns

Aspiration of gastric contents

CONTRAINDICATIONS

Hypoxic patient

During emergency (cardiac arrest) or elective intubations, always ventilate patient with O_2 via face mask and breathing bag before attempting intubation.

Known cervical spine injury

Emergency airway should be established with cricothyroidotomy to avoid the head extension required for endotracheal intubation.

EQUIPMENT (see Appendix for sample kit)

General

    Venous access when time permits

    IV solutions

    Suction with suction catheters and Yankauer suction tip

Resuscitation equipment

    Anesthesia machine or Ambu bag with endotracheal tube and face mask connector

    Drugs for resuscitation as required

    Oxygen

Figure 1   Intubation

    Laryngoscope (curved or straight blade)

    Endotracheal tubes (estimated size and one size smaller)

    Stylette for endotracheal tube, malleable

    Basin with sterile water

    Sterile lubricant, water-soluble

    Syringe, 10-ml

    Scissors

    Clamp—straight mosquito

    Oropharyngeal airway

    Succinylcholine chloride, 20 mg/ml, 1½ mg/kg

    Atropine 0.4 mg/ml, usually 0.6 mg in adult

Tube fixation

    Tincture of benzoin

    Adhesive tape, 1-inch

Ventilation equipment

    Depending on needs of patient

Figure 2   **POSITION**

Supine

Neck flexed (cervical spine)   "Sniffing position"

Head extended (atlantooccipital joint)

TECHNIQUE

(For apneic, relaxed patient. Others may require muscle relaxants to perform intubation.)

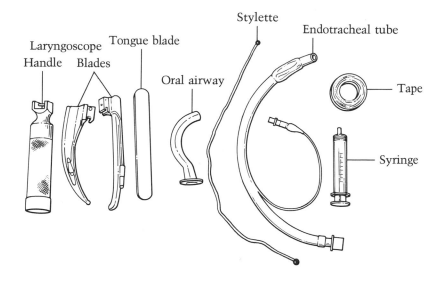

Stylette

Endotracheal tube

Laryngoscope
Handle   Blades   Tongue blade   Oral airway

Tape

Syringe

Figure 1
Intubation equipment.

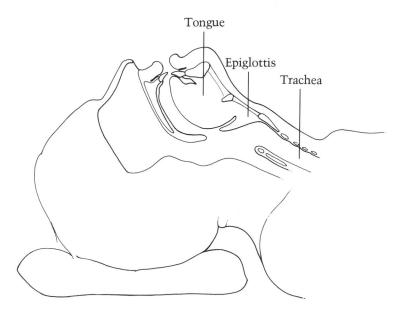

Tongue

Epiglottis

Trachea

Figure 2
Position.

1. Select endotracheal tube

Use soft (low pressure) cuff tube.

Average size:

Adult male	9 mm diameter
Adult female	8 mm diameter
Neonate	3.5 mm diameter
Premature	2.5 mm diameter
Children	Age 5, 5.5 mm diameter
	Each 2 years older: 0.5 mm increase
	Each 2 years younger: 0.5 mm decrease

Select estimated tube size and one next size smaller.

Figure 3

2. Prepare endotracheal tube

Check cuff for leaks by inflating cuff underwater.

Lubricate tube and stylette.

Insert stylette into tube and bend into appropriate curve.

Do not allow stylette to protrude from end of tube.

3. Give atropine

Give 0.6 mg IV in adult.

Omit if has been given as premedication or if emergency demands immediate intubation.

Helps reduce secretions and avoid vagovagal bradycardia.

Figure 4A

4. Insert laryngoscope: curved blade technique

Open laryngoscope, check light.

Open patient's mouth with right hand.

Spread patient's lips to avoid catching them between teeth and laryngoscope blade.

Hold laryngoscope in left hand.

Insert blade between patient's teeth.

Keep to right side of mouth; push tongue to left.

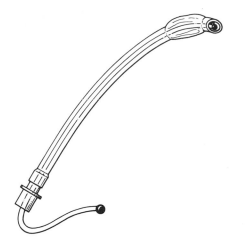

Figure 3
Prepare endotracheal tube.

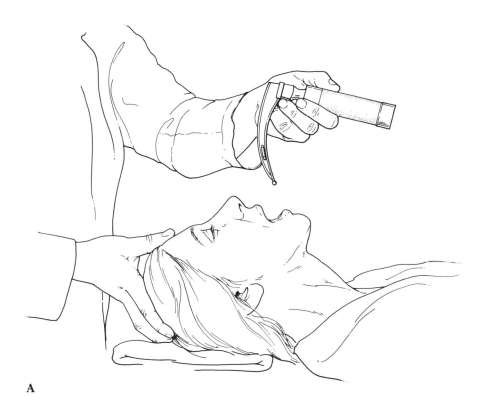

A

Figure 4A
Insert laryngoscope:
curved blade technique.

Figure 4B

Advance blade to groove between base of tongue and epiglottis—do not cover epiglottis with blade.

Lift laryngoscope upward and forward—this elevates base of tongue and epiglottis, bringing larynx into view.

Do not lever laryngoscope.

Do not use teeth as fulcrum.

Figure 5

4A. Insert laryngoscope: straight blade technique

Insert blade into patient's mouth as with curved blade technique.

Advance blade to just beyond tip of epiglottis (dorsal to or covering epiglottis).

Lift laryngoscope upward and forward; then proceed as with curved blade technique.

Figure 6

5. Insert endotracheal tube

Hold in right hand with bevel facing laterally.

Slide gently between cords until proximal end of cuff is immediately below cords.

Remove laryngoscope.

Hold tube stable; remove stylette.

6. Ascertain proper tube position

Hold tube stable.

Attach to positive pressure ventilation bag, 100% oxygen.

Apply intermittent positive pressure.

Ascertain bilateral chest expansion.

Ascertain bilateral equal air entry by auscultation.

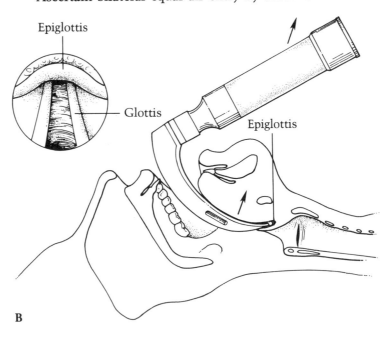

Figure 4B

B

164   17. Endotracheal Intubation

Laryngoscope blade

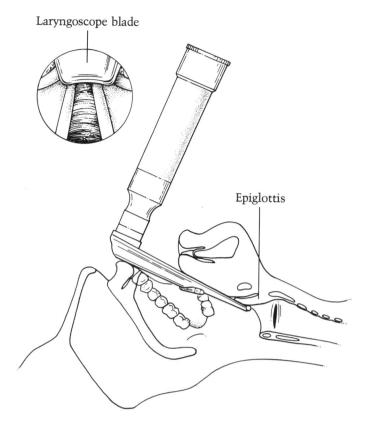

Epiglottis

Figure 5
Insert laryngoscope:
straight blade technique.

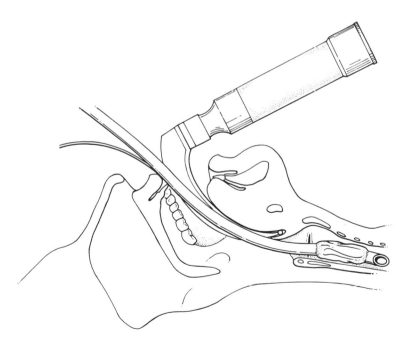

Figure 6
Insert endotracheal tube.

Figure 7

7. Inflate cuff

Inflate just sufficiently to stop reflux around tube (listen at mouth) as positive pressure ventilation is applied.

4 ml air is usually maximum in adult.

Clamp cuff inflation tube distal to observation balloon.

Figure 8

8. Secure endotracheal tube

Cut endotracheal tube so that no more than 3 cm protrudes beyond lips.

Insert oropharyngeal airway.

Apply tincture of benzoin to cheeks.

Tape tube at level of exit from mouth and securely to cheeks.

9. Connect tube to appropriate ventilation device

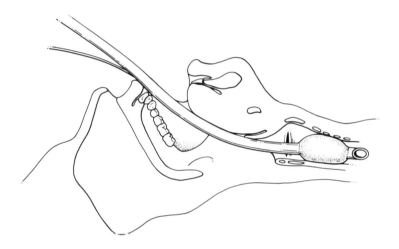

Figure 7
Inflate cuff.

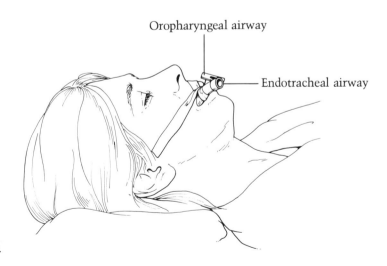

Oropharyngeal airway

Endotracheal airway

Figure 8
Secure endotracheal tube.

EXTUBATION

1. **Suction pharynx to remove secretions**

2. **Suction endotracheal tube**

   Limit suctioning to 10 seconds.

   Unneccessary if no secretions

3. **Ventilate patient**

   Use breathing bag, 100% oxygen.

   Give several deep breaths.

4. **Remove tube**

   Deflate cuff.

   Withdraw tube after deep inspiration.

   Apply face mask delivering oxygen.

COMPLICATIONS

Local trauma

Etiology

   Excessive roughness causing laceration of lips, gums, tongue, pharynx, vocal cords, or trachea.

   Laryngoscope used as a lever with upper teeth as fulcrum, dislodging teeth.

Prevention

   Insert gently and with adequate visualization.

   Do not use laryngoscope as lever.

Cardiac arrhythmias

Etiology

   Increased vagal or sympathetic stimulation in presence of hypoxia or hypercarbia.

Prevention

   Avoid hypoxia and hypercarbia by adequate preoxygenation and ventilation.

Aspiration of gastric contents

Etiology

   Vomiting or passive reflux of gastric contents with aspiration.

Prevention

   Avoid prolonged mask ventilation (with risk of gastric distention) when possible.

Avoid pressure on abdomen during intubation (increases intragastric pressure).

Intubate expeditiously—repeated attempts in awake patient may lead to vomiting.

Esophageal intubation

Etiology

Inadequate visualization of cords with consequent blind intubation and esophageal entry.

Prevention

Properly visualize cords.

Bronchial intubation

Etiology

Tube pushed too far beyond cords, usually entering the right main stem bronchus.

Prevention

Advance tube only until cuff is immediately below cords.

Tape tube securely at this position. Do not place tape distally on tube, but directly as it leaves mouth

Note: Other complications are related to the presence of the dwelling endotracheal tube rather than the intubation procedure itself. Some of the most important are glottic edema, tracheomalacia, and tracheal stenosis. Refer to bibliography for more detailed information.

SELECTED BIBLIOGRAPHY

1. Collins, V. J. *Principles of Anesthesiology* (2d ed.). Philadelphia: Lea & Febiger, 1976. P. 379.

   Complete classification of complications of intubation.

2. Intubation of the Trachea. In R. Dripps et al., *Introduction to Anesthesia* (4th ed.). Philadelphia: Saunders, 1972. Pp. 186–199.

   Step-by-step description of the techniques of tracheal intubation and complications.

3. Magill, I. V. Endotracheal anesthesia. *Am. J. Surg.* 34:450, 1936.

   The "father of modern endotracheal intubations" gives an account of his design of an endotracheal tube and the technique of intubation.

4. Waters, R. M., Rovenstine, E. A., and Guedel, A. E. Endotracheal anesthesia and its historical developments. *Anesth. Analg.* (Cleve.) 12:196, 1933.

   Good historical and developmental account of intubation and the improvement of inhalational anesthetic technique.

18.
Cricothyroidotomy for Emergency Airway

Method of Bruce S. Cutler

INDICATIONS

Emergency airway when endotracheal intubation is unsuccessful

Oropharyngeal airway obstruction due to trauma or foreign body

Note: Cricothyroidotomy is an emergency airway procedure, quicker and safer than tracheostomy under urgent conditions outside the operating room. It is not recommended for use in lieu of the standard tracheostomy, which should always be performed under controlled circumstances in the operating room. Although the incidence of subglottic stenosis is reported to be low, long-term follow-up on a large series of patients is not available.

EQUIPMENT (see Appendix for sample kit)

Skin prep

    Sterile sponges

    Acetone-alcohol solution

    Povidone-iodine solution

Sterile field

    Mask, gown, gloves

    Towels

    Basin with sterile water

    Fenestrated drape

    Towel clips, 4

Local anesthetic

    Syringe, 10-ml

    Needle, 22-gauge × 1½-inch

    Lidocaine 1%, 10 ml

Tracheostomy equipment

> #3 knife handle
>
> #11 scalpel blade
>
> Delaborde dilator
>
> Assortment of standard size tracheostomy tubes (soft cuff)
>
> Crile hemostats, 2
>
> Needle holder
>
> Sutures, 0 silk on curved cutting needle, 2
>
> Catgut ties, 2-0
>
> Suction equipment and tracheal suction catheters
>
> Plastic syringe, 10-ml

POSITION

Figure 1

Supine, head of bed elevated 15 degrees

Rolled towel under shoulders

Neck hyperextended

TECHNIQUE

1. Prep and drape the neck

2. Use mask, gown, and gloves

3. Examine tracheostomy tube

Check cuff for leaks by inflating under water.

Confirm that obturator fits cannula.

Figure 2

4. Identify anatomical landmarks

Palpate cricothyroid space.

Steady thyroid cartilage between thumb and forefinger.

5. Infiltrate local anesthetic

Infiltrate transversely across cricothyroid membrane.

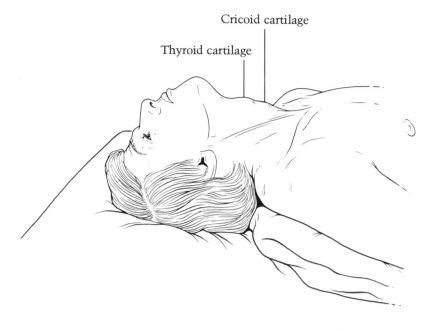

Cricoid cartilage

Thyroid cartilage

Figure 1
Position.

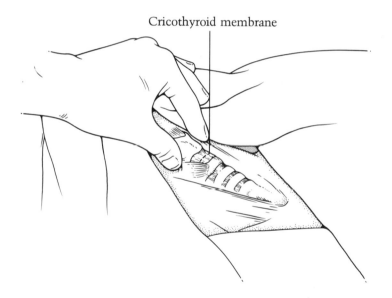

Cricothyroid membrane

Figure 2
Identify anatomical land-
marks.

Figure 3

6. Incise cricothyroid membrane

Puncture skin and cricothyroid membrane with scalpel blade to enter trachea.

Extend incision 1 cm in each direction.

Figure 4

7. Insert Delaborde dilator

Insert dilator along knife blade.

Remove blade.

Figure 5

8. Insert tracheostomy tube

Spread dilator.

Insert tracheostomy tube with obturator.

Remove dilator.

Remove obturator.

Immediately suction trachea.

Ventilate patient via tracheostomy tube.

Figure 6

Inflate cuff with minimum pressure to overcome airway leak.

9. Secure tracheostomy tube

Suture wings of tracheostomy tube to skin.

Tie umbilical tapes to slot at each side of tracheostomy tube.

Tie free ends together around patient's neck.

Dress with sterile sponge under flanges of tracheostomy tube.

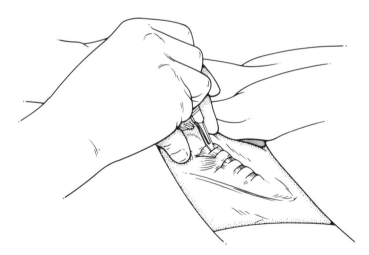

Figure 3
Incise cricothyroid membrane.

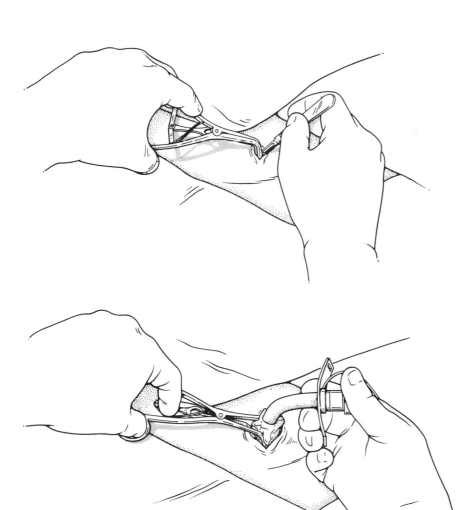

Figure 4
Insert Delaborde dilator.

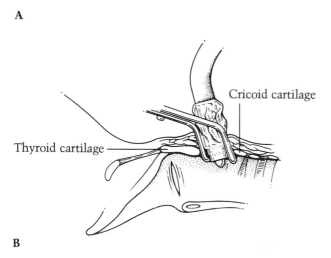

A

Cricoid cartilage

Thyroid cartilage

B

Figure 5
Insert tracheostomy tube.

10. Removal of tube

(Tube may be removed or changed at any time after placement.)

Suction trachea.

Cut umbilical tape and sutures.

Deflate cuff.

Remove tube.

Cover incision with sterile dressing.

COMPLICATIONS

Intraoperative bleeding

Etiology

Laceration of venous plexus.

Prevention

Incise directly over cricothyroid membrane.

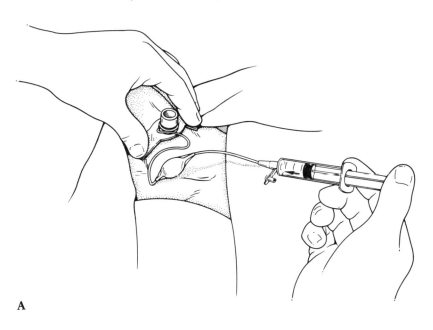

A

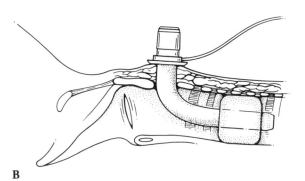

Figure 6
Inflate cuff.

B

Late bleeding

Etiology

Erosion of tube into subcutaneous vessel.

Tracheoinnominate artery fistula from cuff erosion.

Prevention

Subcutaneous vessel erosion may be unavoidable; control with packing or direct suture.

Avoid tracheoinnominate fistula by using low pressure cuff tube.

Tracheostomy tube does not enter trachea

Etiology

Incision too small; tracheostomy tube too large for trachea.

Prevention

Make adequate incision; spread dilator widely; ascertain that tracheostomy tube is smaller than tracheal lumen.

Cuff rupture

Etiology

Overinflation of cuff, laceration of cuff during placement.

Defective cuff.

Prevention

Check cuff for leaks before use.

Ascertain that tracheostomy tube is of appropriate size for tracheal lumen.

Avoid instrument contact with balloon.

Treatment

Replace tracheostomy tube.

Air leakage past tracheostomy tube

Etiology

Insufficient air in cuff; ruptured cuff.

Prevention

Select appropriate size tracheostomy tube for tracheal lumen.

Inflate balloon with minimal amount of air to overcome leak.

If cuff is ruptured, replace tracheostomy tube.

Tracheostomy tube occluded

Etiology

Overinflation of cuff (with herniation of balloon over tube); tracheostomy tube plugged with secretions.

Prevention

Do not overinflate cuff.

Inflate cuff with minimal amount of air to overcome leak.

Suction patients as needed.

Use heated humidity to help prevent mucous concretions.

Tracheal stenosis at cuff site

Etiology

Pressure necrosis of trachea from high pressure balloon cuff.

Prevention

Use low pressure type cuff.

Inflate with minimum pressure needed to avoid air leak.

CARE OF TRACHEOSTOMY

Daily

Change dressing, cleanse and dry adjacent skin.

If double cannula tracheostomy tube is used, remove and clean inner cannula 3 times daily.

Weekly

Replace tracheostomy.

As needed

Endotracheal suctioning

SELECTED BIBLIOGRAPHY

1. Brantigan, C. O., and Grow, J. B., Sr. Cricothyroidotomy: Elective use in respiratory problems requiring tracheotomy. *J. Thorac. Cardiovasc. Surg.* 71:72, 1976.

    Description of extensive experience with 655 cricothyroidotomies.

2. Head, J. M. Tracheostomy in the management of respiratory problems. *N. Engl. J. Med.* 264:587, 1961.

    Discussion of indications and complications of tracheostomy.

3. Safar, P., and Penninckx, J. Cricothyroid membrane puncture with special cannula. *Anesthesiology* 28:943, 1967.

    Description of use as emergency airway procedure.

4. Sercer, A. Tracheostomy through two thousand years of history. *Ciba Symp.* 10:78, 1962.

    Scholarly review of the history of tracheostomy.

5. Stemmer, E. A., Oliver, C., Carey, J. P., et al. Fatal complications of tracheotomy. *Am. J. Surg.* 131:288, 1976.

    Review of fatal tracheotomy complications in 36 patients.

19.
Thoracentesis

Method of
Thomas J. Vander Salm

INDICATIONS

Diagnosis of pleural effusion

Therapeutic removal of pleural air or liquid

EQUIPMENT (see Appendix for sample kit)

Skin prep

    Sterile sponges

    Acetone-alcohol solution

    Povidone-iodine solution

Sterile field

    Gloves, mask

    Fenestrated drape

Local anesthetic

    Syringe, 5-ml Luer-Lok

    Needles

        25-gauge × ⅝-inch

        22-gauge × 2-inch

    Lidocaine 1%, 10 ml

Thoracentesis

    Syringes

        50-ml plastic Luer-Lok

        5-ml Luer-Lok

Needles

22-gauge × 2-inch

18-gauge × 2-inch

15-gauge × 2-inch

Stopcock, 3-way

Curved clamps, 2

Rubber tubing attached to stopcock sidearm

Specimen bowl

Specimen tubes, 3 with stoppers

Optional

14-gauge Intracath

Syringe, 10-ml non-Luer-Lok

Sterile intravenous tubing

Plasma vacuum bottle

Dressing

Sterile sponges

Adhesive tape, 1-inch

POSITION

Figure 1

Air removal

Supine

Head of bed elevated 30–45 degrees

Figure 2

Liquid removal

Sitting

Arms supported on bedside table

TECHNIQUE

1. Review current erect chest x-ray

Confirm diagnosis, location, and extent of pleural air or liquid.

Acute respiratory insufficiency (e.g., tension pneumothorax, rapidly developing effusion) may demand thoracentesis without x-ray.

2. Use mask and gloves

3. Prep and drape

Figure 1

Air removal

Use second or third intercostal space, midclavicular line, to avoid internal mammary artery.

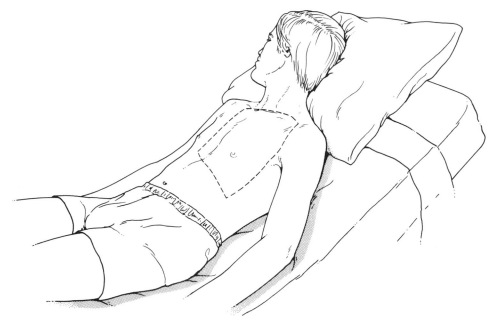

Figure 1
Position for air removal.

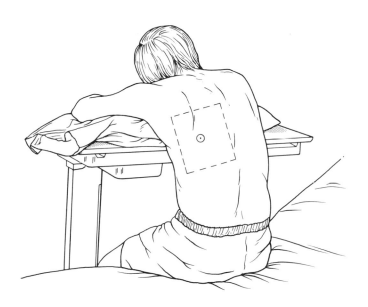

Figure 2
Position for liquid removal.

179

Figure 2

Liquid removal

Confirm fluid level by dullness to percussion; use first or second interspace below in posterior axillary line but not lower than eighth intercostal space.

Figure 3

4. Infiltrate local anesthetic and confirm presence of air or fluid

Inject at superior margin of rib to avoid intercostal bundle.

Infiltrate through pleura (a "give" or "pop" is often felt).

Aspirate to confirm presence of air or fluid.

Mark needle depth with clamp and withdraw needle.

Figure 4A

5. Insert thoracentesis needle (on syringe) to same depth as that marked by clamp

Interpose 3-way stopcock between 15-gauge needle (for liquid) or 18-gauge needle (for air) and 50-ml plastic Luer-Lok syringe.

Mark needle depth with second clamp to prevent excessive penetration.

Figure 4B

Insert needle in same tract to same depth as that marked by clamp.

Do not open needle to atmosphere through stopcock.

6. Aspirate specimen

Use sidearm of 3-way stopcock for effluent specimen.

7. Remove needle, apply sterile dressing

8. Send specimen for studies as appropriate

Cell count

Gram stain

Culture

Cytology and cell block

Protein, sugar, amylase

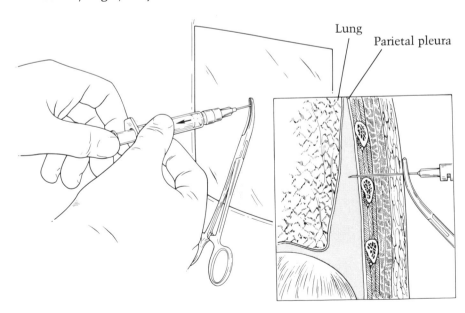

Figure 3
Infiltrate local anesthetic; confirm presence of air or fluid.

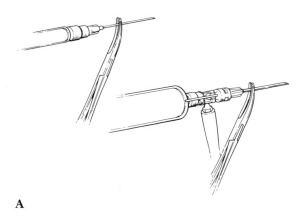

A

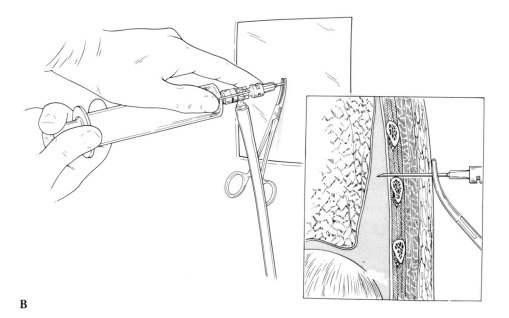

B

Figure 4
Insert thoracentesis needle
(on syringe) to same depth
as that marked by clamp.

9. Obtain chest x-ray

Confirm amount evacuated.

Check for pneumothorax.

ALTERNATIVE TECHNIQUE: FOR TENSION PNEUMOTHORAX

Immediately insert 15-gauge needle in 2d intercostal space, midclavicular line

Place chest tube subsequently.

ALTERNATIVE TECHNIQUE: FOR LARGE FLUID VOLUMES

1–4. Identical to standard procedure

5A. Insert 14-gauge Intracath needle on syringe

Place 10-ml non-Luer-Lok syringe on Intracath needle—no stopcock.

Mark needle depth with second clamp to prevent excess penetration.

Insert needle in same tract to same depth.

Figure 5A, B

6A. Insert cannula through needle

Remove syringe, occlude needle with finger to avoid major pneumothorax, and insert cannula in needle.

Advance cannula into pleural space and slide needle back over cannula.

Never slide cannula back out of needle.

(Cannula previously placed on clamped intravenous tubing attached to plasma vacuum bottle.)

7A. Open tubing clamp to initiate drainage

8A. At completion, remove cannula and needle, and apply sterile dressing

9A. Send specimen for studies as appropriate

Cell count

Gram stain

Culture

Cytology and cell block

Protein, sugar, amylase

10A. Obtain chest film

Check completeness of fluid evacuation.

Check for pneumothorax.

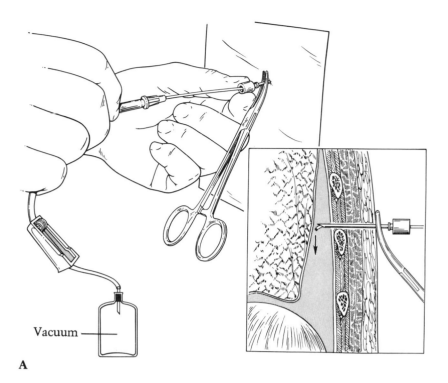

Vacuum

A

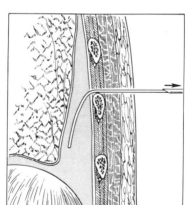

B

Figure 5
Insert cannula through
needle.

COMPLICATIONS

Bleeding

Etiology

Laceration of intercostal vessel.

Prevention

Insert needle at superior margin of rib: major intercostal bundle lies against caudal edge of rib above.

Pneumothorax

Etiology

Inadvertent opening of 3-way stopcock so that pleural cavity is open to atmosphere.

Laceration of lung with needle.

Prevention

Be familiar with stopcock before performing thoracentesis.

Use short-beveled needle.

Insert needle no further than necessary to collect fluid.

Hepatic or splenic puncture

Etiology

Puncture site too caudal and/or too deep.

Prevention

Avoid puncture lower than eighth intercostal space posteriorly.

Mark proper needle depth with clamp to prevent excessive depth of puncture.

SELECTED BIBLIOGRAPHY

1. Bowditch, H. I. Paracentesis thoracis. *Am. J. Med. Sci.* 23:103, 1852.

   First description of the technique in the American literature, but technique credited to Dr. Morrill Wyman.

2. Gott, P. H. A simplified method for thoracentesis and pleural fluid drainage. *Am. Rev. Respir. Dis.* 92:295, 1965.

   Technique of using an Intracath.

3. Hoffmann, L. A modified thoracentesis technique. *Am. Rev. Respir. Dis.* 89:106, 1964.

   Ingenious alternate method of draining large volumes using siphon effect rather than a plasma vacuum bottle.

4. Neptune, W. B. Thoracentesis. In P. F. Nora (ed.), *Operative Surgery*. Philadelphia: Lea & Febiger, 1972. Pp. 217–218.

   Good drawings of the standard technique.

20.
Pleural Biopsy

Method of
Thomas J. Vander Salm

INDICATIONS

Undiagnosed pleural effusion (when thoracentesis nondiagnostic)

Undiagnosed pleural thickening

Particularly useful in the diagnosis of tuberculosis

EQUIPMENT (see Appendix for sample kit)

Skin prep

Sterile sponges

Acetone-alcohol solution

Povidone-iodine solution

Sterile field

Gloves and mask

Fenestrated drape

Local anesthetic

Syringe, 5-ml

Needles

25-gauge × ⅝-inch

22-gauge × 1½-inch

Lidocaine 1%, 10 ml

Figure 1

Biopsy

Scalpel blade, #11

Cope needle (4 parts)

Syringe, 10-ml

Specimen dish with filter paper (sterile)

10% formalin

Dressing

Sterile sponge

Adhesive tape, 1-inch

POSITION

Figure 2

Sitting, arms supported on bedside table

or

Figure 3

Lateral decubitus

(Position varies with intended biopsy site.)

TECHNIQUE

(For biopsy in presence of pleural effusion)

1. Review current chest x-rays

Localize area.

2. Use mask and gloves

3. Prep and drape

Confirm fluid level by dullness to percussion; prep several interspaces above and below.

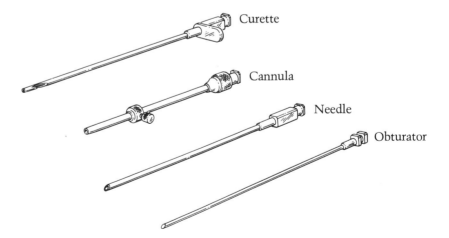

Figure 1
Cope needle.

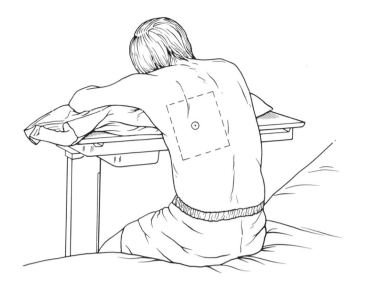

Figure 2
Sitting position.

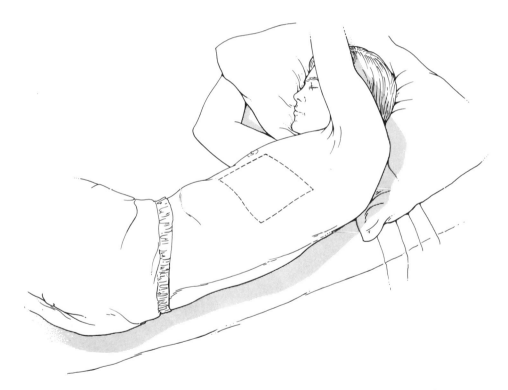

Figure 3
Lateral decubitus position.

Figure 4

4. Infiltrate local anesthetic and aspirate fluid

Inject at superior margin of rib to avoid intercostal bundle.

Do not inject lower than eighth intercostal space in posterior axillary line or seventh intercostal space in anterior axillary line.
Infiltrate to and through pleura.

Aspirate to confirm presence of fluid.

Mark needle depth with clamp, withdraw needle.

Figure 5

5. Incise skin

Use #11 knife blade.

Incise 1–2 mm, on puncture site.

6. Insert Cope cannula

Place obturator in needle; place needle in cannula.

Mark cannula depth with movable sleeve and set screw.

Figure 6A

Insert through anesthetized tract to measured depth.

Figure 6B

Withdraw obturator from needle; replace with 10-ml syringe.

Aspirate to confirm presence of fluid.

Figure 6C

Withdraw needle and cannula slightly until gentle aspiration yields no fluid—this places cannula just external to pleura.

Withdraw needle from cannula.

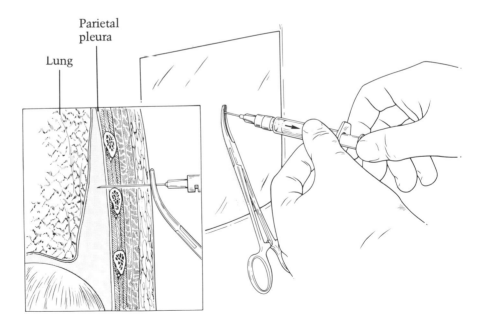

Figure 4
Infiltrate local anesthetic and aspirate fluid.

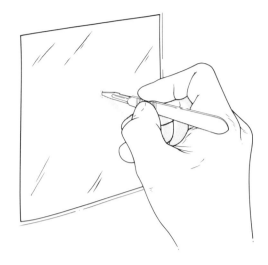

Figure 5
Incise skin.

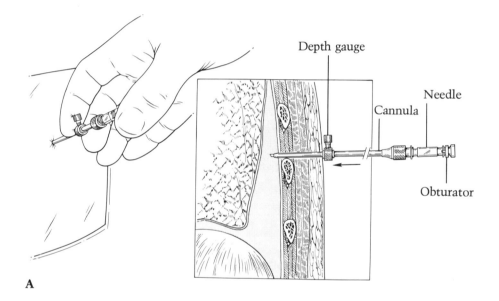

Depth gauge

Needle

Cannula

Obturator

A

Figure 6A
Insert Cope cannula to
measured depth.

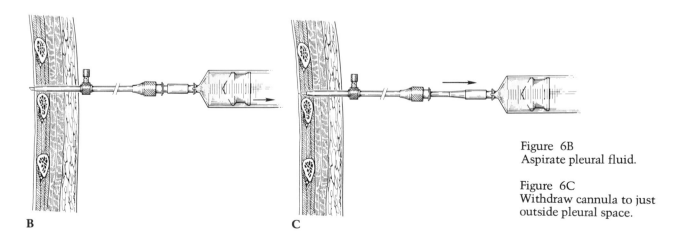

B

C

Figure 6B
Aspirate pleural fluid.

Figure 6C
Withdraw cannula to just
outside pleural space.

7. Perform biopsy

Figure 7A

Place syringe on curette.

Insert curette into cannula until it is within thorax, as determined from fluid aspiration.

(Lip on curette points to biopsy hook—to avoid intercostal bundle, do not biopsy superior quadrant.)

Figure 7B

Withdraw cannula and curette at 10–15-degree angle from that of insertion; engage parietal pleura firmly with hook.

Figure 7C

With curette held stationary, advance cannula with rotating motion to transect specimen held in hook.

Withdraw cannula and curette slightly until cannula is just external to pleura.

Figure 7D

Remove curette, extract specimen.

Biopsy inferior, medial, lateral quadrants.

After last biopsy, remove curette and cannula together.

Place specimens on sterile filter paper in 10% formalin; send for histological examination.

8. Apply sterile dressing

ALTERNATIVE TECHNIQUE

(For biopsy of thickened pleura in absence of pleural fluid)

Procedure similar to foregoing, but absence of pleural fluid makes identification of proper depth more difficult. Care must be taken to avoid lung laceration.

COMPLICATIONS

Hemothorax

Etiology

Bleeding diathesis.

Biopsy of intercostal vessel.

Prevention

Confirm normal clotting status before performing biopsy.

Avoid biopsy in superior quadrant.

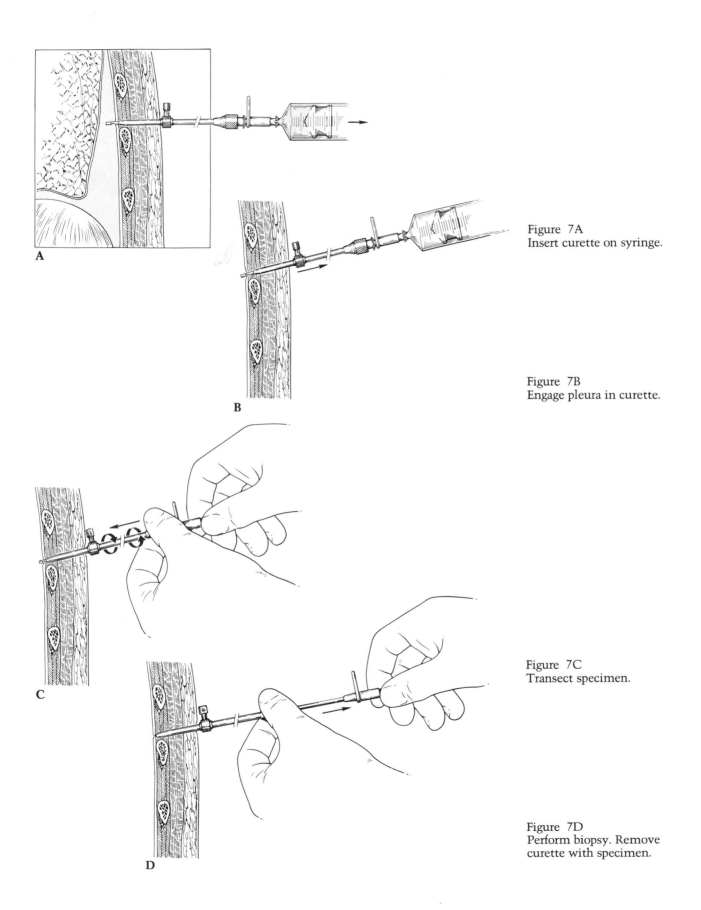

Figure 7A
Insert curette on syringe.

Figure 7B
Engage pleura in curette.

Figure 7C
Transect specimen.

Figure 7D
Perform biopsy. Remove
curette with specimen.

Pneumothorax

Etiology

Aspiration of air through cannula.

Laceration of lung.

Prevention

When cannula is open to air, keep it withdrawn slightly outside pleural space.

Keep syringe on needle or curette when they lie in pleural space.

Avoid deep penetration if procedure is done for thickened pleura in absence of fluid.

Inadequate specimen

Etiology

Bent hook on curette.

Prevention

Inspect hook before use.

Avoid bending hook on rib.

SELECTED BIBLIOGRAPHY

1. Abrams, L. D. A pleural-biopsy punch. *Lancet* 1:30, 1958.

   Description of the punch biopsy instrument designed by Abrams while at the Harefield Hospital in Middlesex (and thus often called a Harefield needle). Widely used, especially in Europe.

2. Cope, C. New pleural biopsy needle. *J.A.M.A.* 167:1107, 1958.

   First description of the needle bearing the author's name. Good descriptive drawing.

3. DeFrancis, N., Klosk, E., and Albano, E. Needle biopsy of the parietal pleura. *N. Engl. J. Med.* 252:948, 1955.

   First description of needle biopsy of the pleura, the Vim-Silverman needle being used.

4. Kettel, L. J., and Cugell, D. W. Pleural biopsy. *J.A.M.A.* 200:317, 1967.

   Good description of technique, indications, and complications of the procedure.

5. Rao, N. V., Jones, P. O., Greenberg, S. D., et al. Needle biopsy of parietal pleura in 124 cases. *Arch. Intern. Med.* 115:34, 1965.

   Indicates the wide range of diagnoses made with pleural biopsy and the early stage at which tuberculosis is often diagnosed.

6. Scerbo, J., Keltz, H., and Stone, D. J. A prospective study of closed pleural biopsies. *J.A.M.A.* 218:377, 1971.

   Study showing that closed pleural biopsy may be performed in the absence of pleural effusion.

21.
Chest Tube Insertion (Closed Thoracostomy)

Method of Thomas J. Vander Salm

INDICATIONS

Removal of air or liquid from pleural space

Instillation of chemotherapeutic agent after removal of malignant effusion

EQUIPMENT (see Appendix for sample kit)

Skin prep

    Sterile sponges

    Acetone-alcohol solution

    Povidone-iodine solution

Sterile field

    Gloves, mask

    Fenestrated drape

Local anesthetic

    Syringe, 10-ml

    Needles

        25-gauge × ⅝-inch

        21-gauge × 1½-inch

    Lidocaine 1%, 20 ml

Tube insertion

  Knife handle

  #10 scalpel blade

  Curved clamp (Rochester-Pean)

  Chest tube—type and size depend on purpose and preference

    Pneumothorax

      Adults: #24 Fr. Argyle straight

      Infants: #18 Fr. Argyle straight

      Children: Progressively larger size with larger children

  Tubing and connectors (to fit tubing and chest tube)

    Hemothorax or pleural effusion

      Adults: #32 Fr. Argyle straight or right angle

      Infants: #20 Fr. Argyle straight or right angle

      Children: Largest tube consistent with child's size

  3-bottle chest suction

  Needle holder

  Skin suture, 2-0 silk

  Suture scissors

Dressing

  Petrolatum gauze

  Sterile sponges

  Tincture of benzoin

  Elastoplast, 4-inch

  Adhesive tape, 1-inch

POSITION

Figure 1   Anterior apical tube

  Supine

  Head of bed elevated 30–45 degrees

Figure 2   Basilar or lateral apical tube

  Lateral decubitus, involved side up

TECHNIQUE: PNEUMOTHORAX

1. Use gloves and mask

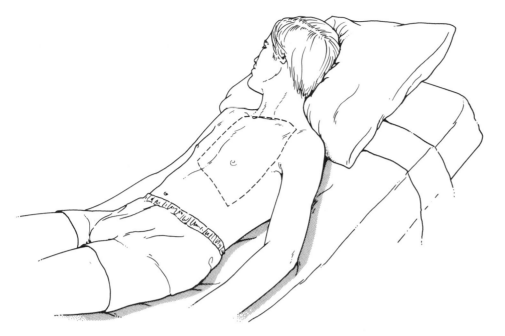

Figure 1
Position for anterior apical
tube.

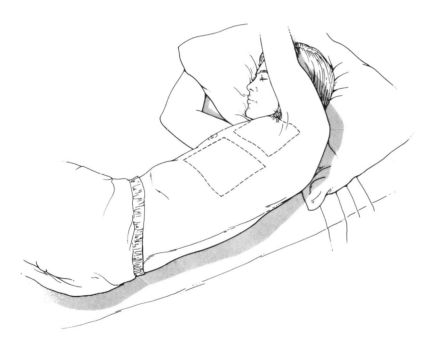

Figure 2
Position for basilar or lateral apical tube.

Figure 1

2. Prep and drape

Second or third intercostal space, midclavicular line, to avoid internal mammary artery

Alternative site

Midaxillary line, caudal edge of axillary hair line

For cosmetic reasons in women

For technical reasons in muscular men with thick pectoralis major

Figure 3

3. Infiltrate local anesthetic; aspirate to confirm pneumothorax

Infiltrate desired interspace to pleura and aspirate to confirm pneumothorax.

In order to permit tunneling of tube, infiltrate skin over next caudal interspace.

Note: Chest tube insertion is often very painful without adequate local anesthesia: in adults 1% lidocaine, 20 ml, is often needed.

Figure 4A, B

4. Incise skin; create tunnel

Make incision one intercostal space caudal below that of pleural entry and large enough to admit little finger (smaller in infants and small children).

Create tunnel by spreading clamp.

Figure 5

5. Perforate into pleural space

Grip clamp along shaft to prevent plunging too deeply into chest.

Perforate endothoracic fascia and pleura at top edge of rib.

Spread clamp to enlarge hole; remove clamp.

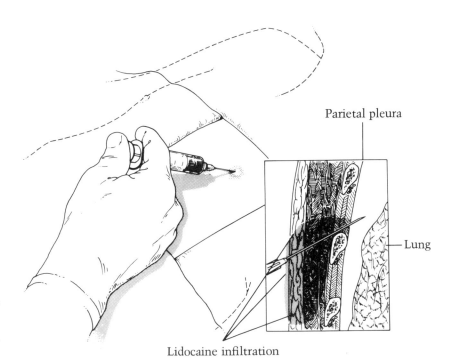

Parietal pleura

Lung

Lidocaine infiltration

Figure 3
Infiltrate local anesthetic, aspirate to confirm pneumothorax or hemothorax or pleural effusion.

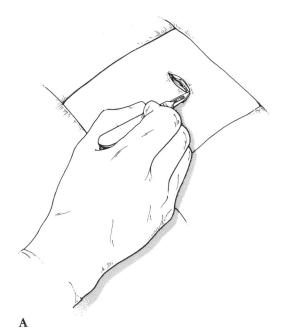

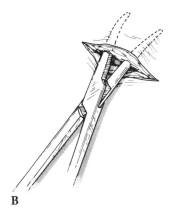

Figure 4A
Incise skin.

Figure 4B
Create tunnel.

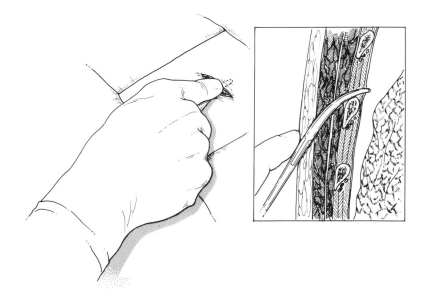

Figure 5
Perforate into pleural
space.

Figure 6

6. Explore pleural space (except in infants and small children)

Use fifth finger to

Assure tract large enough for tube.

Guard against extrapleural tube placement.

Confirm free pleural space.

Figure 7

7. Insert chest tube

Grasp chest tube with clamp.

Guide into pleural space.

Advance tube to apex; leave no holes external to pleural space.

Air whistling to and fro in tube indicates proper intrapleural placement but creates open pneumothorax.

Figure 8

8. Quickly attach chest tube to 3-bottle water-seal suction

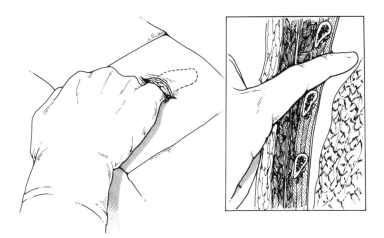

Figure 6
Explore pleural space.

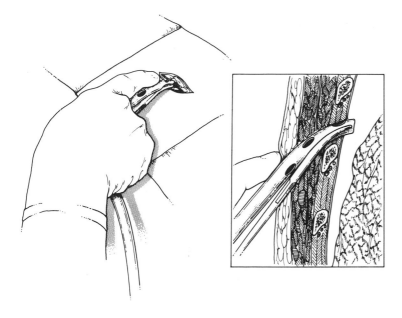

Figure 7
Insert chest tube.

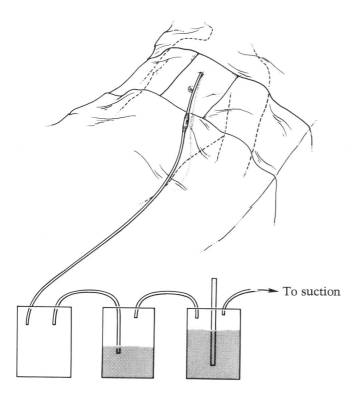

To suction

Figure 8
Attach chest tube to 3-bottle water-seal suction.

Figure 9

9. Suture skin, secure chest tube

Leave one suture long and tie *securely* around chest tube.

In infants, also place horizontal mattress suture and leave untied for closing tract when tube is removed.

Figure 10

10. Apply dressing

Apply tincture of benzoin to skin.

Place petrolatum gauze around tube exit site so as to make airtight seal.

Cover with dry sterile dressing and Elastoplast.

Further secure chest tube with adhesive tape.

11. Tape all chest tube connections

12. Obtain chest x-ray

Assess position of chest tube and for resolution of pneumothorax.

TECHNIQUE: HEMOTHORAX OR PLEURAL EFFUSION

1. Use gloves and mask

Figure 2

2. Prep and drape

Place tube dependently, in fluid.

Use sixth or seventh intercostal space, midaxillary line, unless fluid is loculated elsewhere.

Tube should not enter posterior to midaxillary line; patient will lie on tube, causing discomfort and kinking of the tube.

Figure 3

3. Infiltrate local anesthetic; aspirate to confirm hemothorax or pleural effusion

Infiltrate desired interspace to pleura, and aspirate to confirm fluid.

In order to permit tunneling of tube, infiltrate skin over next caudal interspace.

Note: Chest tube insertion is often very painful without adequate local anesthesia: in adults, 1% lidocaine, 20 ml, is often needed.

4–6. Same as for pneumothorax

7. Insert chest tube

Grasp tube with clamp.

Guide into pleural space.

Advance posteriorly and basally; leave no holes external to pleural space.

Figure 8

8. Attach to 3-bottle chest suction

Figures 9, 10

9. Same as for pneumothorax

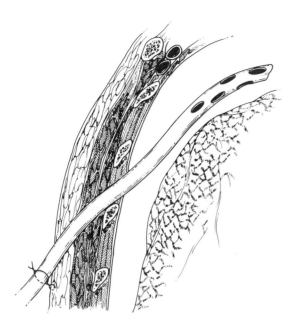

Figure 9
Suture skin, secure chest tube.

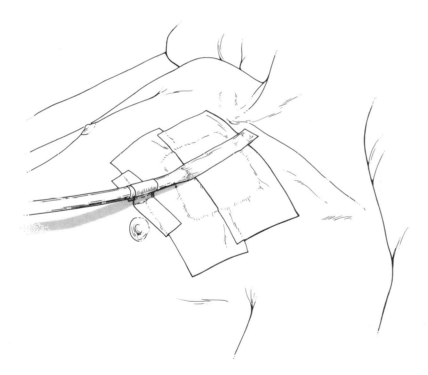

Figure 10
Apply dressing.

ALTERNATIVE PROCEDURES

The foregoing techniques are generally applicable.

Many variations in techniques and tubes are available.

Pneumothorax: Foley catheter technique

Insert Foley catheter through a trocar.

Inflate balloon and pull it back against the chest wall as catheter is sutured in place.

Pneumothorax: emergency one-way valve

Cut a finger from a rubber glove and tie it over external end of chest tube.

Cut a small hole in end of glove finger to create a one-way valve.

Chest tube variations

Argyle plastic chest tubes are available with indwelling stylette, permitting use as a large (but potentially dangerous) trocar.

COMPLICATIONS

Laceration of lung

Etiology

Plunging instrument into chest, injuring lung parenchyma or pulmonary vessels.

Prevention

Aspirate at proposed interspace to confirm presence of air or liquid.

Grip instrument so that distance from hand to tip is just greater than chest wall thickness (see Figure 5).

Chest wall bleeding

Etiology

Laceration of intercostal or internal mammary vessels.

Prevention

Insert instruments or tubes along top edge of rib to avoid intercostal vessels.

Place anterior tubes not closer to sternum than midclavicular line.

Improper position of tube

Etiology

Blind placement.

Prevention

Find proper tract with finger exploration to avoid lung, adhesions, or extrapleural position.

Air leak into chest tube system

Etiology

Loose connectors.

Chest tube holes external to pleural space.

Broken chest tube bottles.

Prevention

Firmly tape all connections.

Position all chest tube holes in pleural cavity.

Check chest tube bottles before using.

Chest tube occlusion

Etiology

Blood clots or viscous pleural effusion.

Kinking of chest tube.

Prevention

Strip chest tubes hourly: compress between two rollers of chest tube stripper and manually push contents of tube distally.

Insert sufficiently large tube; for hemothorax in adults, #28 is minimum.

Insert additional tube to help evacuate blood if needed.

Eliminate kinking by proper positioning and exit location of the tube—never place tube posterior to midaxillary line.

Persistent pneumothorax

Etiology

Large air leak with failure of lung to expand.

Treatment

Increase suction.

Large air leak may require surgical closure.

Consider placing second chest tube if question exists as to proper function or placement of first tube.

Subcutaneous emphysema

Etiology

Pneumothorax inadequately decompressed by chest tube may cause air to leak into subcutaneous space if skin is tightly sealed around chest tube.

Prevention

If subcutaneous emphysema increases progressively, enlarge space between skin and chest tube to vent subcutaneous space.

If subcutaneous emphysema is stable, no treatment is necessary.

CHEST TUBE REMOVAL

EQUIPMENT (see Appendix for sample kit)

Sterile sponges, 4-inch × 4-inch

Petrolatum gauze

Scissors

Elastoplast, 4-inch

Tincture of benzoin

POSITION

Supine

TECHNIQUE

1. **Remove dressing and tape from chest wall**

    Removal from chest tube unnecessary

2. **Instruct patient**

    Tell patient to breathe deeply with forced expiration against pursed lips.

    Reassure that procedure is painless.

Figure 11   3. **Cut suture anchoring chest tube**

Figure 12   4. **Apply dressing**

    Tincture of benzoin to surrounding skin

    Petrolatum gauze, then sterile dry sponge over incision

5. **Remove tube**

    While patient practices forced expiration through pursed lips, rapidly slide chest tube out of chest.

    Maintain steady pressure on dressing.

    In infants and small children, tie previously placed horizontal mattress suture.

6. **Apply occlusive dressing**

7. **Obtain chest x-ray**

    Check for induced pneumothorax.

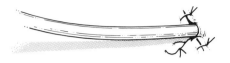

Figure 11
Cut suture anchoring
chest tube.

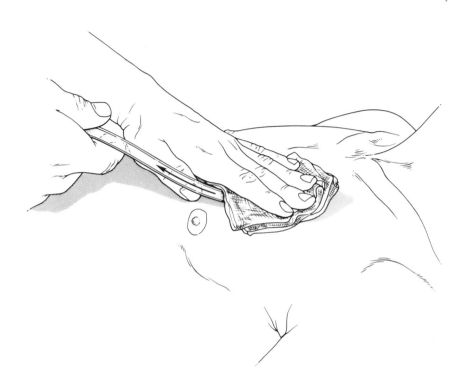

Figure 12
Apply dressing, remove
tube.

205

COMPLICATIONS

Pneumothorax

Etiology

> Air leaking in around tube or through holes in side of tube that are extrathoracic while others still lie intrathoracic.

Prevention

> Ensure positive intrapleural pressure.

> Valsalva maneuver accomplishes this best, but some patients gasp at the time of tube removal, thus creating negative intrapleural pressure. The compromise measure of expiration against pursed lips reduces tendency to gasp.

> Remove tube rapidly.

> Keep firm pressure on dressing; particularly important in children, who are especially likely to develop a pneumothorax on tube removal.

> Tunneling of tube during insertion produces oblique tract, with decreased likelihood of air entry.

Blood on operator's clothing

Prevention

> Wear gown, stand to side when pulling tube out.

SELECTED BIBLIOGRAPHY

1. Kovarik, J. L., and Brown, R. K.   Tube and trocar thoracostomy. *Surg. Clin. North Am.* 49:1455, 1969.

   Good description of the technique.

22.
Control of Epistaxis

Method of
Thomas J. Vander Salm
and Richard R. Gacek

INDICATIONS

Epistaxis

EQUIPMENT (see Appendix for sample kit)

Inspection

    Emesis basin

    Headlight (or head mirror with light source)

    Bayonet forceps

    Nasal speculum

    Nasal suction (#5 Fraser tip)

    Cotton pledgets

Topical anesthetic

    Cotton pledgets

    Cocaine, 4%

Anterior epistaxis control

    Cautery

        Silver nitrate sticks

        or

        Electric cautery

    Nasal pack—selvage gauze, ½-inch or 1-inch

    Surgicel gauze

    Neosporin ointment

    Suture scissors

Posterior epistaxis control

Gloves

Catheters, 2 flexible, #12–14 Fr.

Umbilical tape

Neosporin ointment

Petrolatum gauze, 3-inch × 36-inch

Dental roll

Two Rochester-Pean clamps, 7-inch

POSITION

Sitting, head supported, facing examiner

PREPARATION

Figure 1A, B

Review anatomy

Kiesselbach's plexus on anterior septum is site of 90% of epistaxis.

Obtain brief history

Trauma usually indicates anterior epistaxis.

Blood first appearing in pharynx usually indicates posterior epistaxis.

Bleeding disorders, hypertension, and nasal tumors require additional treatment.

TECHNIQUE FOR DETERMINATION OF BLEEDING SITE

1. Adjust headlight

Figure 2

2. Inspect nose

Open nostril with nasal speculum.

Remove blood with suction tip.

Continued bleeding demonstrates side of nosebleed.

3. Determine site of bleeding

Anterior epistaxis or epistaxis from under turbinates usually can be directly visualized with aid of suction.

Posterior epistaxis cannot be visualized directly but can be demonstrated by resumption of bleeding as suction tip advances beyond bleeding point.

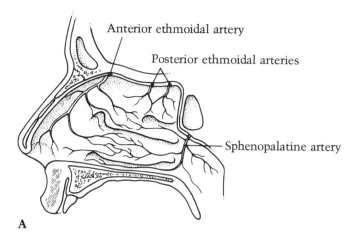

A

Figure 1
Anatomy. A. Nasal ala.

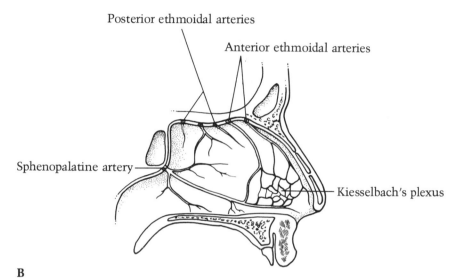

Posterior ethmoidal arteries

Anterior ethmoidal arteries

Sphenopalatine artery

Kiesselbach's plexus

B

B. Nasal septum.

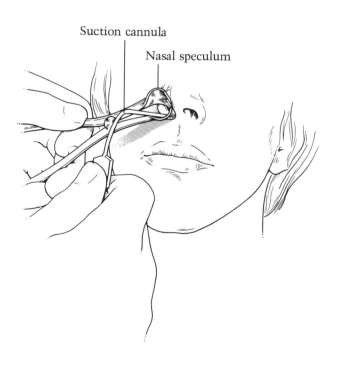

Suction cannula

Nasal speculum

Figure 2
Inspect nose to determine
bleeding site.

209

TECHNIQUE FOR CONTROL OF ANTERIOR BLEEDING

Figure 3

1. Apply local pressure

Insert 4% cocaine-soaked cotton pledget into nostril.

Apply pressure by compressing nasal alae 10 minutes. (Pressure plus cocaine vasoconstriction usually stops anterior epistaxis.)

If bleeding is from under turbinates, pack infraturbinate area with Surgicel before applying pressure.

2. Cauterize bleeding point

Cauterize even if bleeding stopped in step above.

Use silver nitrate stick or electric cautery.

If bleeding persists, or bleeding area large, insert anterior pack.

3. Insert anterior pack

Impregnate selvage gauze with Neosporin ointment.

Figure 4

Insert pack with doubled end to avoid free end working into pharynx.

Figure 5

Fold layers into nose from roof to floor.

Leave pack in place 2–3 days.

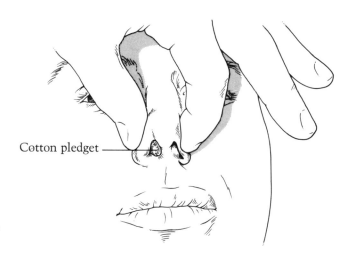

Cotton pledget

Figure 3
Insert cotton pledget
(cocaine-soaked) and apply
pressure.

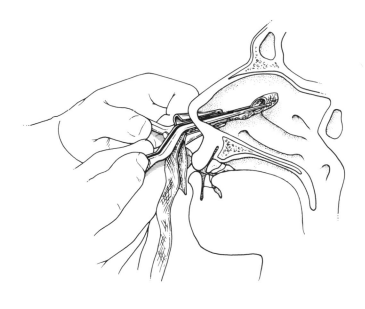

Figure 4
Insert anterior pack.

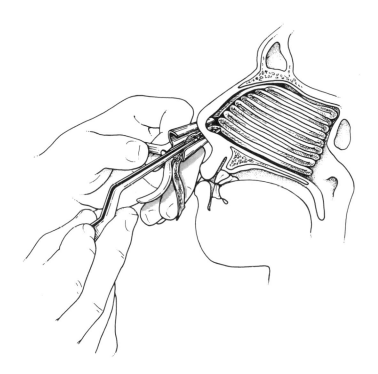

Figure 5
Fold pack in layers.

TECHNIQUE FOR CONTROL OF POSTERIOR BLEEDING

(Patients with posterior packs require hospitalization because of possible respiratory embarrassment.)

Figure 6

1. Prepare posterior pack

Roll 3-inch × 36-inch petrolatum gauze into tight cylindrical pack, 3 inches long.

Tie 18-inch umbilical tape around middle of roll; leave ends long.

Tie second umbilical tape around middle of roll; leave ends long.

Impregnate pack with Neosporin ointment.

2. Insert pack

Thread flexible catheter through nonbleeding side of nose, pull tip from pharynx and out of mouth.

Clamp two ends together.

Thread second flexible catheter through bleeding side of nose, pull tip from pharynx and out of mouth.

Clamp two ends together.

Figure 7

Tie both ends of one umbilical tape around catheter tip from bleeding side.

Pull catheter and umbilical tape back through nose; leave second umbilical tape hanging out of mouth for subsequent removal.

Pull soft palate forward with remaining catheter to facilitate passage of pack.

Figure 8

Pull pack through pharynx into posterior nose, pushing around soft palate with finger.

3. Insert anterior pack (see Technique for Control of Anterior Bleeding, steps 1–3)

Figure 9

4. Secure posterior pack

Tie umbilical tapes over a dental roll against nares.

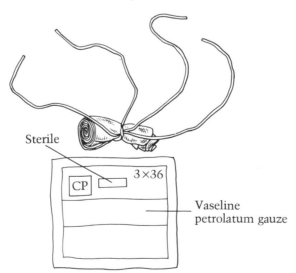

Sterile

CP   3×36

Vaseline petrolatum gauze

Figure 6
Prepare posterior pack.

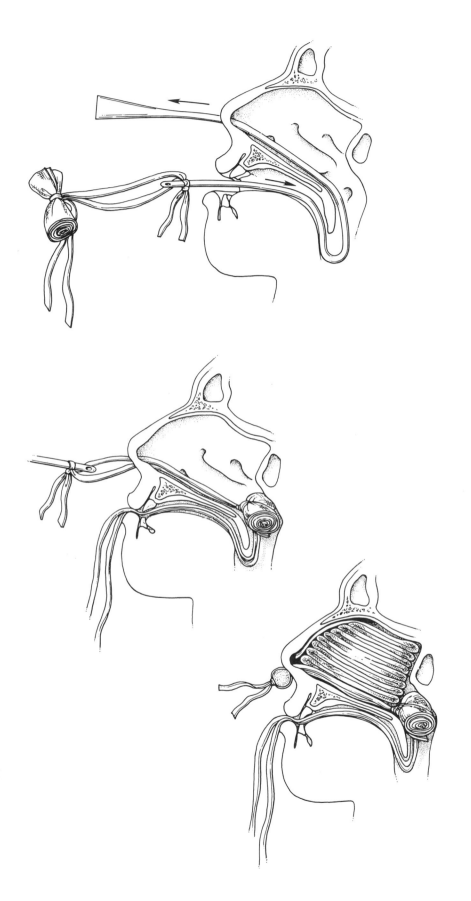

Figure 7
Tie posterior pack to
catheter.

Figure 8
Pull pack into position.

Figure 9
Secure posterior pack by
tying over dental roll.

5. Place patient on oral decongestant and antibiotic

6. Pack removal

Leave posterior pack in 3–4 days; anterior pack 2 days.

Remove anterior pack.

Cut umbilical tapes tied around dental roll.

Using remaining umbilical tapes, gently extract pack from nose and withdraw through mouth.

7. If bleeding resumes

Repack.

Consult ENT surgeon and consider possible vessel ligation (external carotid, internal maxillary, or anterior ethmoidal artery).

COMPLICATIONS

Rhinitis

Etiology

Common with anterior packing.

Occlusion of drainage, mucosal trauma, and bacterial overgrowth.

Prevention

Impregnate pack with topical antibiotic ointment.

Remove anterior pack in 2–3 days; posterior in 4 days.

Maxillary and frontal sinusitis

Etiology

Occlusion of sinus orifices by anterior pack with bacterial overgrowth.

Prevention

Impregnate pack with antibiotic ointment.

Use oral decongestants to reduce secretions.

Use routine systemic antibiotics.

Hemotympanum

Etiology

Blood forced up eustachian tube during bleeding with egress prevented by posterior pack.

Prevention

Not possible, but resolves spontaneously with pack removal.

Otitis media

Etiology

Occlusion of eustachian tube orifice by posterior pack with subsequent bacterial overgrowth.

Prevention

Leave pack in no more than 4 days.

Impregnate pack with antibiotic ointment.

Use oral decongestants to help improve drainage.

Bacteremia

Etiology

Trauma to bacteria-covered mucous membranes during packing.

Prevention

Insert packs gently.

Impregnate packs with antibiotic ointment.

Respiratory embarrassment

Etiology

Sedation.

Impaired airway.
    More common with posterior packs.

Prevention

Hospitalize patients with posterior packs for observation.

Avoid bilateral posterior packs.

Do not oversedate.

Columellar and alar necrosis

Etiology

Repeated packing.

Excessive pressure against mucous membrane.

Prevention

If packing unsuccessful after two tries, proceed to vessel ligation.

Avoid undue pressure against nares.

Cocaine toxicity

Etiology

Overdosage, manifested as CNS stimulation leading to seizures, respiratory failure, sympathetic stimulation (indirect) and, from large doses, direct cardiac toxicity.

Prevention

Limit total topical dose to less than 200 mg in average adult (much less is needed for procedure described here).

Have immediately available:

Rapid-acting intravenous barbiturate.

Capability for mechanical ventilation.

SELECTED BIBLIOGRAPHY

1. Beinfield, H. H.   General principles in treatment of nasal hemorrhage. *Arch. Otolaryngol.* 57:51, 1953.

   Good reference for general management of epistaxis.

2. Hallberg, O. E.   Severe nosebleed and its treatment. *J.A.M.A.* 148:355, 1952.

   Detailed description of method of posterior packing with excellent illustration.

3. Hara, H. J.   Severe epistaxis. *Arch. Otolaryngol.* 75:258, 1962.

   Good general paper on causes and treatment of epistaxis.

4. Herzon, F. S.   Bacteremia and local infections with nasal packing. *Arch. Otolaryngol.* 94:317, 1971.

   Documents clear reduction in bacterial overgrowth on nasal packs when topical antibiotic used, and the 12% incidence of bacteremia associated with use of the pack.

5. Saunders, W. H.   Practical management of nosebleeds. *G.P.* 17:100, 1958.

   Good description of the method of locating the site of bleeding.

6. Smith, R.   Managing epistaxis. *Postgrad. Med.* 55:143, 1974.

   Excellent paper on the management of epistaxis with good drawings of the techniques involved.

23.
Nasogastric Tube Insertion

Method of
Thomas J. Vander Salm

INDICATIONS

Aspiration of gastric contents

Gastric feeding or lavage

EQUIPMENT (see Appendix for sample kit)

Tube preparation

Water-soluble lubricant

Nasogastric tube

For aspiration, Salem sump

For feeding only, small soft tube or Intracath, 36-inch

Tube insertion

Emesis basin

Glass of water with straw

Crushed ice in basin

Syringe, 50-ml catheter tip

Tube fixation

Adhesive tape, 1-inch

Figure 1

POSITION

Sitting

Neck slightly flexed

TECHNIQUE

Figure 2

1. **Estimate distance tube is to be inserted**

   Hold nasogastric tube in curve approximately that of nose, pharynx, esophagus, and stomach, usually 50 cm in adults.

2. **Prepare tube for insertion**

   Apply slight caudal curve to tip.

   Lubricate distal 15 cm of tube.

3. **Slide tube through nose into pharynx**

Figure 3

   Use most patent nostril.

   Instill small amount of lubricant directly into nose.

   Slide tube horizontally to avoid impingement on nasal turbinates.

4. **Slide tube into esophagus as patient swallows**

   Concurrently instill water through tube

   or

   Allow patient to drink water through a straw.

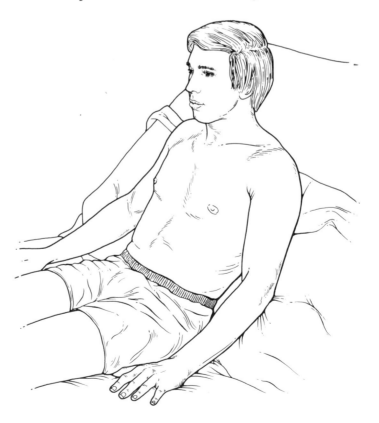

Figure 1
Position.

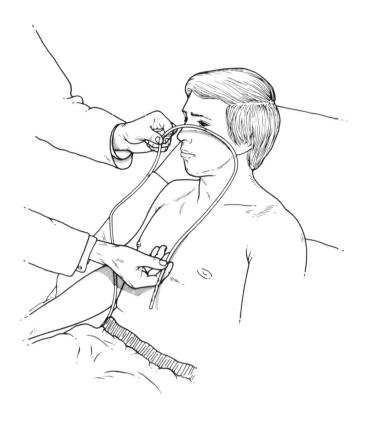

Figure 2
Estimate distance to insert
tube.

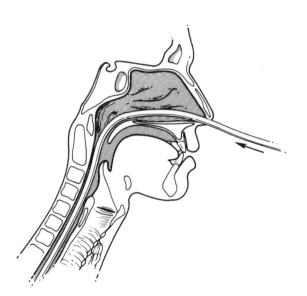

Figure 3
Slide tube into pharynx.

219

Figure 4

5. Position tube in stomach

Insert to predetermined distance.

Auscultation over stomach during injection of 50 ml air into tube confirms intragastric location of tube by characteristic bubbling sound.

Aspiration of gastric contents further confirms position.

Figure 5

6. Tape tube to nose

ALTERNATIVE PROCEDURES

Stiffen soft tube

To avoid curling in pharynx, stiffen tube by cooling with ice.

Pass tube with carrier tube

With very flexible, small tube, wedge tube into gelatin capsule along with stiffer tube to facilitate passage into stomach.

Remove carrier tube after gelatin capsule dissolves.

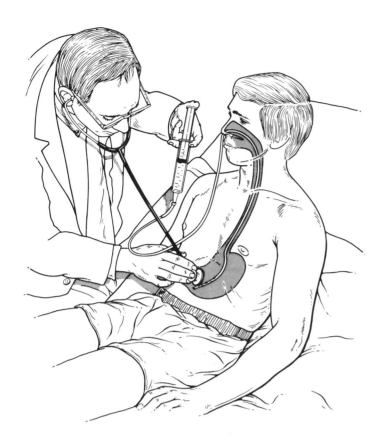

Figure 4
Position tube in stomach.

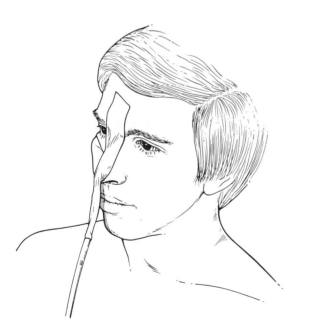

Figure 5
Tape tube to nose.

COMPLICATIONS

Nasotracheal intubation

Etiology

Obtunded patient with poor cough reflex.

Diagnosis

Hoarseness, cough, air efflux from tube, and lack of gastric bubbling with air injection.

Prevention

Withdraw tube, twist 180 degrees, reinsert.

Keep patient's neck flexed.

When possible, ensure swallowing during insertion—this causes epiglottis to close larynx.

Epistaxis

Etiology

Excessive force during insertion of tube, causing tube to lacerate mucous membranes.

Inadequate lubrication.

Prevention

Insert tube in horizontal plane (see Technique, step 4).

Inspect nose initially to ensure adequate patency.

Insert gently.

Lubricate tube well.

Esophageal erosion

Etiology

Prolonged pressure against esophageal wall by firm tube.

Gastroesophageal reflux caused by tube traversing the lower esophageal sphincter.

Prevention

Remove tube as soon as possible.

Use soft tube if prolonged use anticipated.

Gastric bleeding

Etiology

Excessive suction applied to gastric mucosa.

Prevention

Use Salem sump tube to prevent excessive suction and mucosal trauma.

Nasal erosion

Etiology

Pressure on nasal ala from tube.

Prevention

Do not tape tube firmly against nasal ala.

Otitis media

Etiology

Edema at eustachian tube orifice caused by trauma from nasogastric tube.

Prevention

Remove tube as soon as possible.

Spray topical decongestants into nose to treat.

Excessive gagging

Etiology

Hypersensitive gag reflex or emotionally labile patient.

Prevention

Explain procedure to patient.

Do not discuss nausea or vomiting.

Encourage deep breathing (panting) through mouth after tube passes.

SELECTED BIBLIOGRAPHY

1. Kaminski, M. V., Jr. Tube Feeding. EATON Laboratories, 1973.
    Booklet describing technique.
2. ROCOM, Medical Skills Library, Medex International, Inc., Products. Nasogastric Intubation.
    Good visual demonstration of technique (videotape).

24.
Sengstaken-Blakemore Tube Insertion

Method of Thomas J. Vander Salm

INDICATIONS

Continued bleeding *documented* to be from esophageal varices

Massive, uncontrolled upper GI bleeding *likely* to be from esophageal varices

Note: Patient must *be under constant surveillance while tube is in place.*

EQUIPMENT (see Appendix for sample kit)

Tube preparation

    Sengstaken-Blakemore tube (SB tube)

    Nasogastric tube (NG tube), #18

    Syringe, 50-ml to fit SB tube openings

    Water-soluble lubricant

Tube insertion

    Emesis basin

    Glass of water with straw

    Y connector

    Connecting tubing

    Manometer (from sphygmomanometer)

    Bulb inflator (from sphygmomanometer)

    Clamps, 4 Rochester-Pean

Tube fixation

    Adhesive tape, 1-inch

    5-cm cube of foam rubber, cut halfway through

Emergency deflation

    Large scissors

POSITION

Figure 1

Sitting, or, if in shock, supine with head elevated

TECHNIQUE

Figure 2

1. **Mark nasogastric (NG) and Sengstaken-Blakemore (SB) tubes**

   Marks should align two tubes so that NG tube tip is positioned just above esophageal balloon.

2. **Check function of both gastric and esophageal balloons and gastric tube**

3. **Lubricate SB tube; deflate both balloons**

Figure 3

4. **Insert SB tube via nostril into stomach**

   Use most widely patent nostril; if tube too large for nostril, insert perorally.

   Slide SB tube along floor of nose to avoid turbinates.

   When tube is in nasopharynx, advance it into esophagus as patient swallows water.

Figure 4

5. **Confirm position of gastric balloon in stomach**

   Advance to beyond 50-cm mark in adults.

   Irrigate gastric tube with air; auscultate over stomach to confirm position of end of tube.

   (Where possible, fluoroscopic control may be used to avoid gastric balloon inflation in esophagus.)

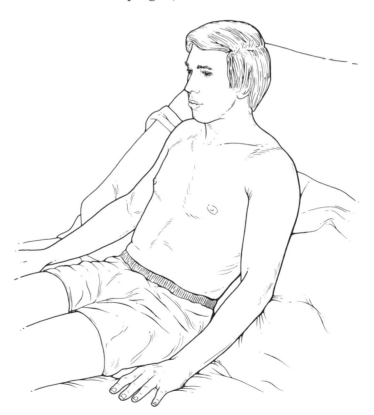

Figure 1
Figure 1
Position.

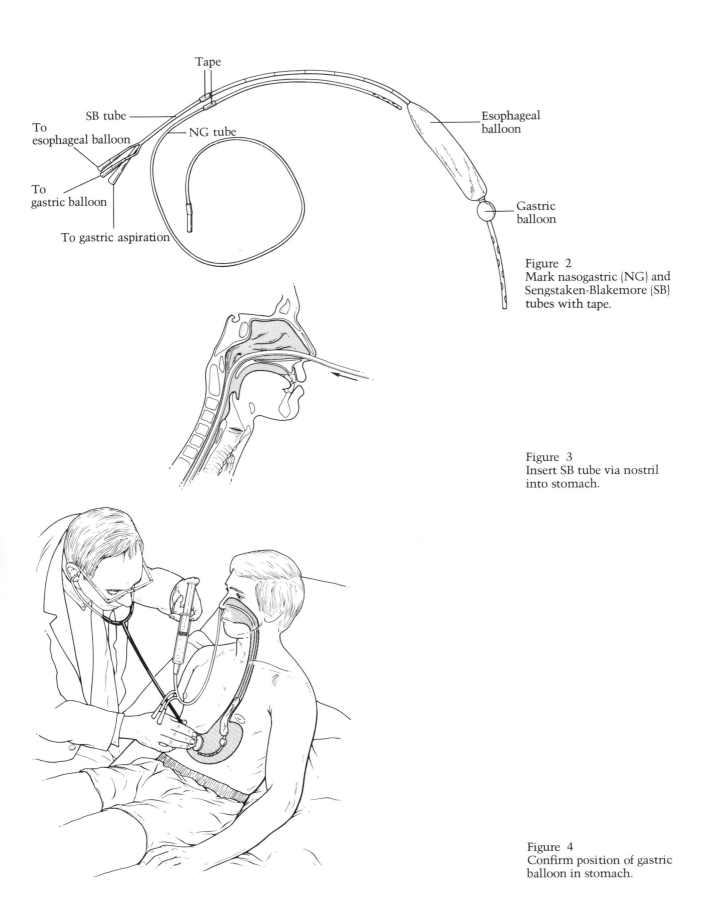

Tape

SB tube

To
esophageal balloon

NG tube

To
gastric balloon

To gastric aspiration

Esophageal
balloon

Gastric
balloon

Figure 2
Mark nasogastric (NG) and
Sengstaken-Blakemore (SB)
tubes with tape.

Figure 3
Insert SB tube via nostril
into stomach.

Figure 4
Confirm position of gastric
balloon in stomach.

Figure 5

6. Inflate gastric balloon

Use 200–250 ml air.

Doubly clamp gastric balloon tube.

Figure 6

Gently pull tube back to seat balloon against gastroesophageal junction.

Secure by applying foam rubber cube around tube as it emerges from nose.

Tape cube to tube, thus supplying gentle traction.

7. Begin gastric suction

Gastric lavage should be performed frequently enough to keep stomach free of clots.

Figure 7

8. Insert nasogastric tube into esophagus and attach to suction

Insert transnasally to previously measured depth.

Alternatively, tie NG tube to SB tube prior to insertion. Increased overall size then demands peroral insertion.

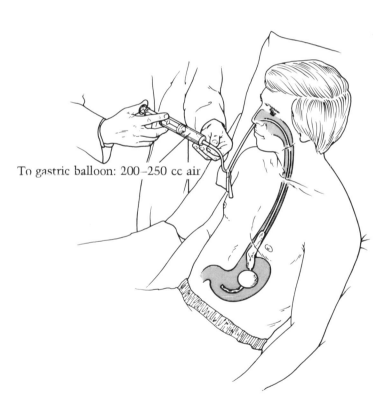

To gastric balloon: 200–250 cc air

Figure 5
Inflate gastric balloon.

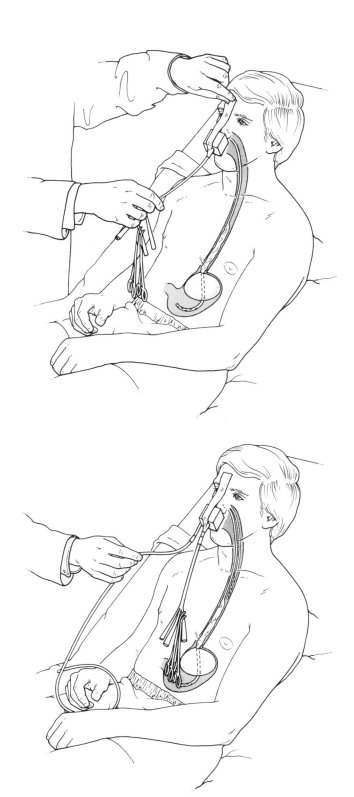

Figure 6
Seat balloon against gas-
troesophageal junction and
secure.

Figure 7
Insert nasogastric tube into
esophagus and attach to
suction.

Figure 8

9. Inflate esophageal balloon

Attach Y connector to esophageal balloon opening.

Attach syringe to one sidearm of Y connector and manometer to other.

Inflate esophageal balloon to 30 mm Hg.

Up to 45 mm Hg may be used if necessary to control bleeding.

Doubly clamp tubing.

Recheck pressure every hour.

10. Tape scissors to head of bed

Airway occlusion may occur if esophageal balloon is pulled into hypopharynx.

Figure 9
Emergency treatment is to cut the SB tube to deflate all balloons, and remove tube.

COMPLICATIONS

Aspiration

Etiology

Vomiting during procedure.

Overflow of blood or secretions from above esophageal balloon.

Prevention

Begin gastric suction soon after SB tube inserted.

Apply suction to blind esophageal pouch to prevent accumulation of blood or secretions.

If endotracheal intubation required, perform before SB tube insertion.

Figure 9

Airway occlusion

Etiology

Obstruction of hypopharynx by inflated esophageal balloon.

Prevention

Ascertain proper position of gastric balloon.

Assure adequate volume in gastric balloon to anchor tube in stomach.

Keep patient under constant observation.

If airway obstruction occurs, transect entire tube immediately with scissors to deflate all balloons. Hold tube between nose and transection point, remove tube.

Never use weights to maintain traction; their use risks pulling the esophageal balloon into the hypopharynx.

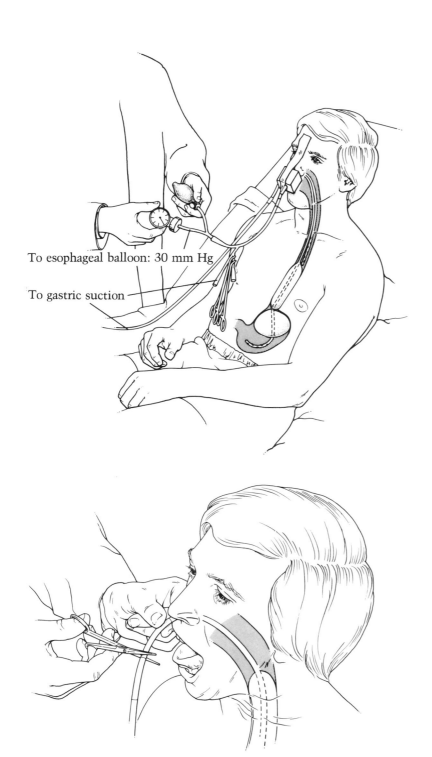

To esophageal balloon: 30 mm Hg

To gastric suction

Figure 8
Inflate esophageal balloon.

Figure 9
Cut tube for airway occlusion.

Esophageal erosion

Etiology

Pressure of balloon against esophageal wall.

Prevention

Remove tube within 48 hours.

Rupture of esophagus

Etiology

Inflation of gastric balloon in esophagus.

Prevention

Carefully confirm location of gastric balloon in stomach before inflation. Auscultation while instilling air into gastric tube is usually sufficient; radiographic control of balloon inflation is better.

Erosion of gastroesophageal junction

Etiology

Prolonged or excessive pressure against gastroesophageal junction.

Prevention

Remove tube within 48 hours.

Use only gentle traction on tube via the foam rubber cube.

Never use weights to apply traction to tube.

SELECTED BIBLIOGRAPHY

1. Blakemore, A. H. Instructions for Passing the Esophageal Balloon for the Control of Bleeding from Esophageal Varices.

   Package insert distributed with SB tube by Davol, Inc.

2. Boyce, H. W., Jr. Modification of the Sengstaken-Blakemore balloon tube. *N. Engl. J. Med.* 267:195, 1962.

   Addition of a nasogastric tube to decompress the proximal esophagus.

3. Conn, H. O., and Simpson, J. A. Excessive mortality associated with balloon tamponade of bleeding esophageal varices: A critical reappraisal. *J.A.M.A.* 202:587, 1967.

   Report of the frequent and often disastrous complications of the use of the SB tube.

4. Pitcher, J. L. Safety and effectiveness of the modified Sengstaken-Blakemore tube: A prospective study. *Gastroenterology* 61:291, 1971.

   Shows the minimization of complications with assiduous attention to details in use of the tube, including the use of the Boyce modification.

5. Sengstaken, R. W., and Blakemore, A. H. Balloon tamponage for the control of hemorrhage from esophageal varices. *Ann. Surg.* 131:781, 1950.

   Original description of the Sengstaken-Blakemore tube and its use.

25.
Cervical Pharyngostomy

Method of
Bruce S. Cutler

INDICATIONS

Prolonged upper gastrointestinal decompression or tube feeding

EQUIPMENT (see Appendix for sample kit)

Skin prep

    Sterile sponges

    Povidone-iodine solution

    Acetone-alcohol solution

Sterile field

    Towels

    Towel clips

    Fenestrated drape

    Gloves

Local anesthetic

    Benzocaine spray, 14% (Cetacaine)

    Topical lidocaine, 4%, 5 ml

    Plastic syringe, 3-ml

    Needle, 22-gauge × 1½-inch

    Injectable lidocaine, 1%, 10 ml

Intubation equipment

    Right angle clamp, 7½-inch

Nasogastric tube

   #14 for feeding

   #16 or #18 for gastric decompression

Knife handle, #3

Scalpel blade, #11

Mayo needle holder

2-0 silk suture on curved cutting needle

Suture scissors

Irrigating syringe, 50-ml

Dressing

   Povidone-iodine ointment

   Sterile sponges

   Tincture of benzoin

   Adhesive tape, 1-inch

Figure 1

POSITION

Head of bed elevated 45–60 degrees

Head turned slightly to opposite side

TECHNIQUE

1. Prep and drape

Figure 2

2. Anesthetize oropharyngeal mucosa in conscious patients

   Have patient gargle for 1 minute with 4% lidocaine.

   Grasp tongue with gauze.

   Spray oropharynx with 14% benzocaine spray.

3. Use gloves

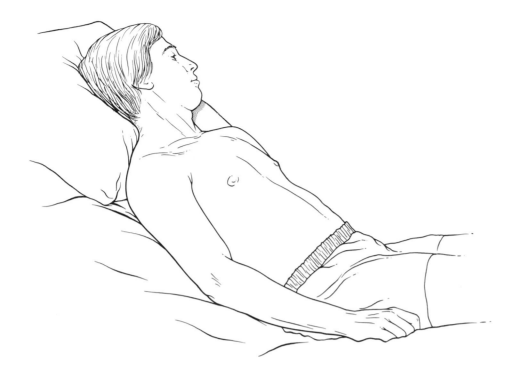

Figure 1
Position, prep, and drape.

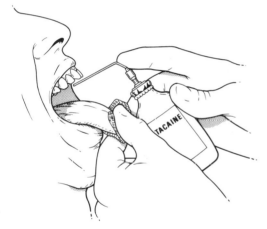

Figure 2
Anesthetize oropharyngeal mucosa in conscious patients.

235

Figure 3

Figure 4

Figure 5

Figure 6

4. Locate pyriform sinus; anesthetize skin

Pass forefinger (right hand for right side) along lateral pharyngeal wall to point just beyond hyoid bone, just medial to greater cornu. This locates the pyriform sinus and is the pharyngostomy site.

Identify this point externally, and infiltrate skin with 1% lidocaine.

5. Perform cervical pharyngostomy

Insert closed right angle clamp through mouth and along lateral pharyngeal wall to point previously palpated.

Palpate clamp tip beyond hyoid bone, medial to greater cornu. At this point, only subcutaneous tissue and thyrohyoid membrane intervene between skin and mucous membrane. Superior thyroid artery lies inferior to intended point of incision.

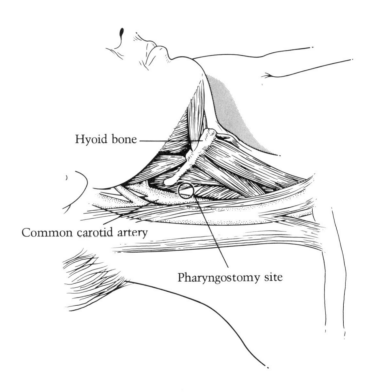

Hyoid bone

Common carotid artery

Pharyngostomy site

Figure 3
Locate pyriform sinus.

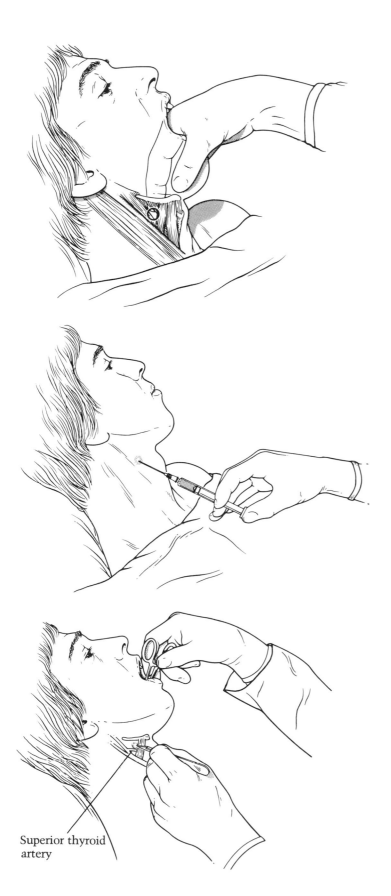

Superior thyroid
artery

Figure 4
Slide finger into pyriform
sinus.

Figure 5
Anesthetize skin over
pyriform sinus.

Figure 6
Perform cervical pharyn-
gostomy.

6. Create tube tract

Figure 6

Make stab wound with #11 blade down to tip of clamp.

Push clamp through to skin surface.

Figure 7

Open jaws of clamp.

Grasp tip of well-lubricated nasogastric tube.

Figure 8

Withdraw approximately 40 cm of nasogastric tube through pharyngostomy into oral cavity.

7. Pass nasogastric tube

Figure 9

Pass nasogastric tube into stomach. (See Chapter 23.)

Confirm intragastric position of tube by auscultation over stomach while insufflating air with irrigating syringe: a characteristic bubbling sound will be heard.

Figure 10

Withdraw excess nasogastric tube through pharyngostomy so that tube passes in smooth curve from pyriform sinus into esophagus.

Recheck position of nasogastric tube by air insufflation while auscultating over stomach.

Suture tube to skin.

8. Apply dressing

Apply povidone-iodine ointment at puncture site.

Apply tincture of benzoin to surrounding skin.

Apply small, secure gauze and adhesive tape dressing.

Tube may be used immediately.

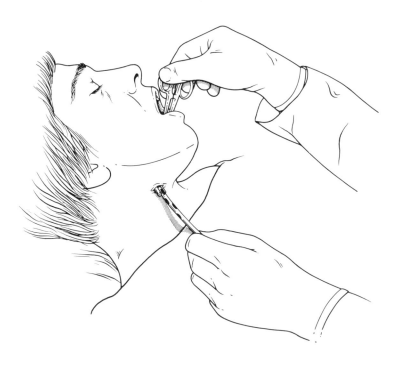

Figure 7
Create tube tract.

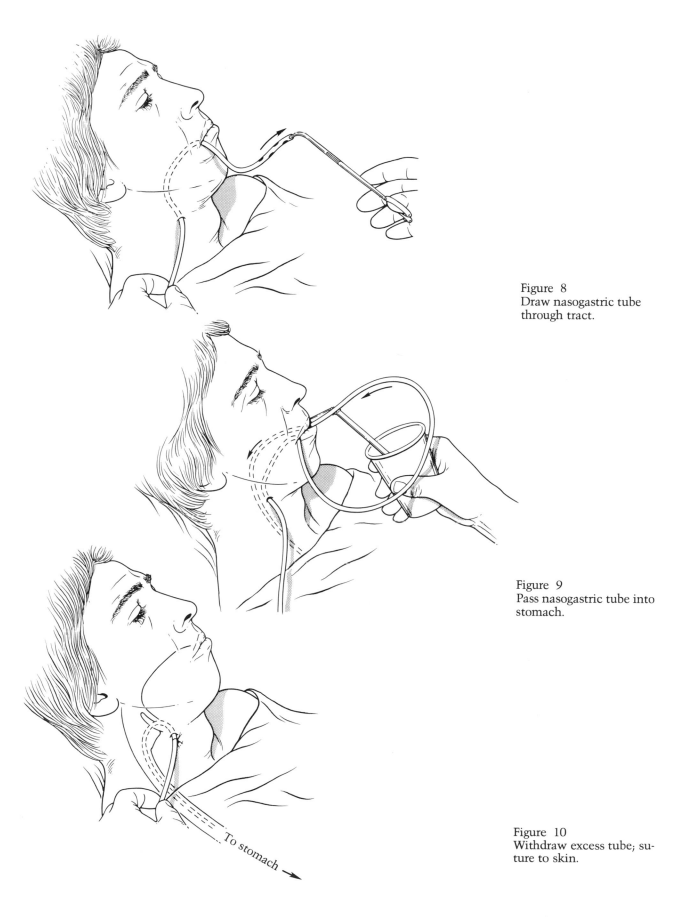

Figure 8
Draw nasogastric tube
through tract.

Figure 9
Pass nasogastric tube into
stomach.

To stomach →

Figure 10
Withdraw excess tube; su-
ture to skin.

239

COMPLICATIONS

Arterial bleeding from puncture site

Etiology

Injury to superior thyroid artery.

Puncture site located too far inferiorly.

Prevention

Position tip of clamp medial to greater cornu of hyoid bone, very close to skin surface, before making incision with knife blade.

Dislodgment of tube

Etiology

Uncooperative patient.

Erosion of suture from prolonged tube placement.

Prevention

Tube may be replaced without difficulty, within several hours of removal, by inserting tip of a well-lubricated nasogastric tube in the sinus tract and instructing patient to swallow as tube is advanced. (See Chapter 23.)

CARE OF CERVICAL PHARYNGOSTOMY TUBE

Daily

Change dressing, inspect suture, and apply povidone-iodine ointment.

Monthly

Change tube, and secure with new suture (as described under Technique).

Removal

Cut suture and remove tube.

Sinus tract will close spontaneously.

SELECTED BIBLIOGRAPHY

1. Lyons, J. H., Jr.   Cervical pharyngostomy. *Am. J. Surg.* 127:387, 1974.

   Excellent technical description.

2. Royster, H. P., Noone, R. B., Graham, W. P., III, et al.   Cervical pharyngostomy for feeding after maxillofacial surgery. *Am. J. Surg.* 116:610, 1968.

   Clinical experience with 55 procedures.

3. Ware, L., Garrett, W. S., Jr., and Pickrell, K.   Cervical esophagostomy: A simplified technique. *Ann. Surg.* 165:142, 1967.

   Technical description with good discussion of complications.

26.
Intestinal Intubation

Method of Bruce S. Cutler

INDICATIONS

Preoperative decompression of mechanical ileus

Instillation of contrast material to diagnose point of obstruction

EQUIPMENT (see Appendix for sample kit)

Figure 1

Intestinal tube (one of the following)

Cantor

Single-lumen, gastrointestinal aspiration only

Kaslow

Single-lumen, gastrointestinal aspiration only

Dennis

Triple-lumen, gastrointestinal sump and mercury instillation

Miller-Abbott

Double-lumen, gastrointestinal aspiration and mercury instillation

Tube preparation

0 silk ligature

Water-soluble lubricant

Metallic mercury, 5 ml

Syringe, 5-ml

Needle, 21-gauge × 1½-inch

Tube insertion

Emesis basin

Water in glass with straw

Irrigation syringe, 50-ml

POSITION

Passage into stomach

Figure 2A

Miller-Abbott or Dennis tube

Sitting, head erect

Figure 2B

Cantor or Kaslow tube

Sitting, neck extended, neck resting on pillow

Passage through pylorus

All tubes

Right lateral decubitus to facilitate passage through pylorus

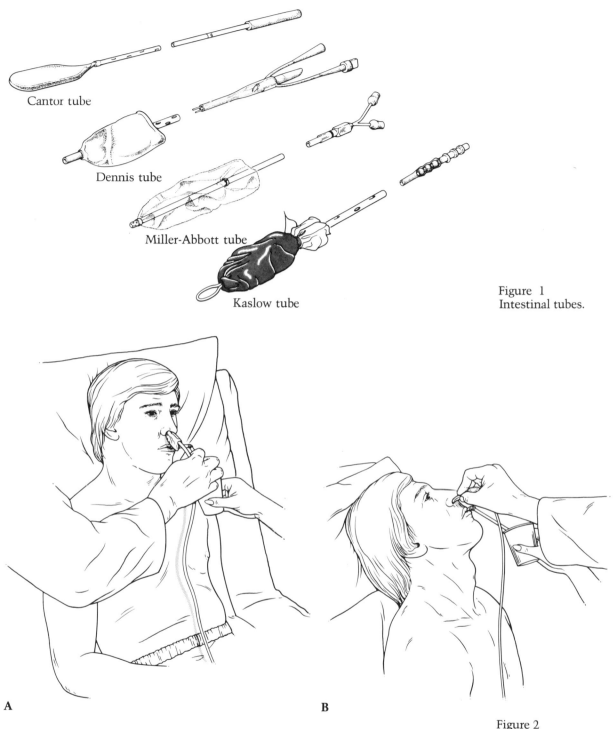

Cantor tube

Dennis tube

Miller-Abbott tube

Kaslow tube

Figure 1
Intestinal tubes.

A

B

Figure 2
A. Miller-Abbott or
Dennis tube. B. Cantor
or Kaslow tube.

TECHNIQUE

1. Prepare tube

Figure 3

Cantor tube

Inject 5 ml mercury into middle of bag, using syringe and 21-gauge needle.

Aspirate all air.

Figure 4

Kaslow tube

Pour 5 ml mercury into proximal end of opened balloon.

Expel all air from balloon.

Tie open end of balloon with strong silk thread.

Figure 5

Trim excess balloon to within 3 cm of tie.

Dennis and Miller-Abbott tubes

Aspirate all air from balloon.

2. Estimate distance to insert tube (distance from nose to stomach and from nose to pylorus)

Hold intestinal tube in curve approximating that of nose, pharynx, and esophagus (usually 50 cm).

Add 15 cm for length of stomach.

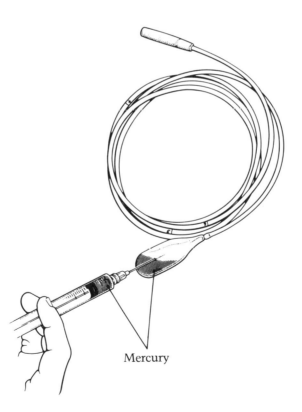

Mercury

Figure 3
Prepare tube: Cantor tube.

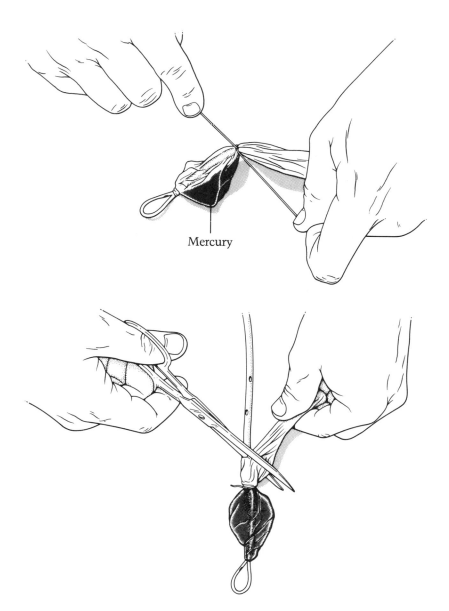

Mercury

Figure 4
Prepare tube: Kaslow tube.

Figure 5
Prepare tube: trim excess
from Kaslow tube balloon.

3. Insert tube into nose

Use most patent nostril.

Lubricate end of tube.

Cantor and Kaslow tubes

Hold tip of catheter so that mercury drops to base of balloon.

Figure 6   Fold balloon lengthwise to trap mercury at base of bag.

Insert tube into nostril.

Figure 7   Release hold on balloon so mercury runs to tip of balloon, drawing it into pharynx.

Dennis and Miller-Abbott tubes

Pass tip of catheter along floor of nose to pharynx.

Figure 8
4. Slide tube into esophagus as patient swallows

Instill water through tube or allow patient to drink water through straw as tube is advanced.

Do not force passage of tube.

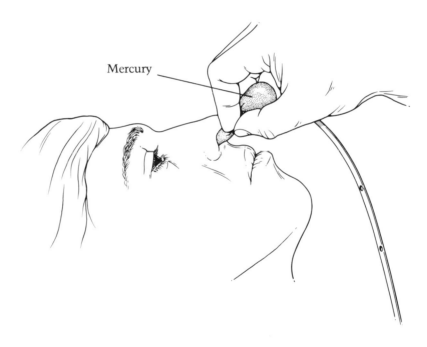

Mercury

Figure 6
Insert tube into nose.

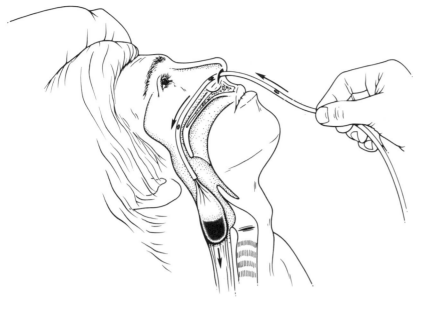

Figure 7
Allow mercury bag to
draw tube into pharynx.

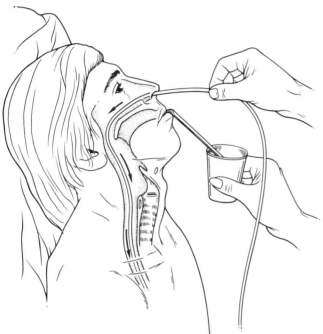

Figure 8
Slide tube into esophagus
as patient swallows.

247

Figure 9

5. **Position tube in stomach**

   Insert to predetermined distance (50 cm) so tip of tube is in stomach.

   Confirm intragastric position by auscultation over stomach during injection of 50 ml of air.

6. **Fill balloon with mercury (Dennis and Miller-Abbott tubes only)**

   Add 2–5 ml mercury through balloon lumen.

7. **Pass tube through pylorus**

   Place patient on right side for 2 hours minimum.

   Slowly advance the tube to the 65-cm mark during this time.

8. **Check position of tube with fluoroscopy**

   Tube may be manipulated under fluoroscopy to facilitate passage through pylorus.

9. **Advance tube when beyond pylorus**

   Connect tube to intermittent gastric suction. (Use continuous suction with Dennis sump tubes.)

   Do not secure tube to nose.

   Allow tube to advance by peristalsis.

   Keep 4 inches of tube outside nose lubricated.

10. **Removal of tube**

    Dennis and Miller-Abbott tubes

      Aspirate mercury before removal.

      Apply slow steady traction.

      Maintain suction, or clamp tube, to prevent aspiration of small bowel fluid during withdrawal.

COMPLICATIONS

Leakage into intestinal lumen

Etiology

   Rupture of balloon.

Prevention

   Use gentle technique during insertion and withdrawal.

   (Metallic mercury is relatively nontoxic; observe to assure passage from bowel.)

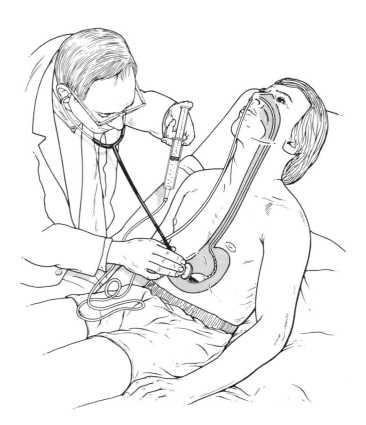

Figure 9
Position tube in stomach.

Tube fails to pass pylorus

Etiology

Coiling of excess tube in stomach.

Prevention

Pass tube only to premeasured mark (65 cm).

Instillation of 500 ml of air into stomach will eliminate redundant gastric folds and may facilitate passage.

Pass tube under fluoroscopic control.

Tube fails to pass into small intestine

Etiology

Absence of peristalsis.

Prevention

Pass tube early in course of intestinal obstruction, before peristalsis ceases.

Place tube on suction during passage to reduce intestinal distention.

SELECTED BIBLIOGRAPHY

1. Miller, L. D., Mackie, J. A., and Rhoads, J. E. The pathophysiology and management of intestinal obstruction. *Surg. Clin. North Am.* 42:1285, 1962.

   Excellent review of the pathophysiology of intestinal obstruction.

2. Miller, T. G., and Abbott, W. O. Intestinal intubation: A practical technique. *Am. J. Med. Sci.* 187:595, 1934.

   Original description of the Miller-Abbott tube.

3. Scheltema, G. Permeation in the examination and treatment of the stomach and intestines. *Arch. Roentgen Ray* 13:144, 1908.

   Amusing account of the earliest therapeutic uses of long intestinal tubes.

4. Smith, B. C. Experiences with the Miller-Abbott tube. *Ann. Surg.* 122:253, 1945.

   Statistical analysis of the Miller-Abbott tube in 1000 cases.

5. Welch, C. *Intestinal Obstruction.* Chicago: Year Book, 1958.

   Excellent description of various types of tubes, indications for intubation, and complications.

27.
Sigmoidoscopy

Method of
Wayne E. Silva

INDICATIONS

Diagnostic

Evaluation or treatment of anal or rectal disease

EQUIPMENT (see Appendix for sample kit)

Positioning

Sigmoidoscopic table or bed

Patient drape

Insertion of sigmoidoscope

Lubricant

Gloves

Inspection

Proctosigmoidoscope, 25–30 cm, with eyepiece, light, obturator, and inflating bulb

Suction

Suction tip cannula with tubing

Suction source

Biopsy

Biopsy forceps

Insulated suction tip and electrocautery

Specimen bottle

10% formalin

Figure 1

BOWEL PREPARATION

Laxative the night before and prepackaged enema ½ to 1 hour before procedure

Contraindicated in patients with massive GI bleeding, diarrhea, or inflammatory bowel disease

POSITION

Figure 2

Head-down position

Best position for examination; proctology table required

Figure 3

Knee-chest position

Poorly tolerated by the elderly and debilitated

Figure 4

Left lateral Sims's position

Most comfortable for obese, elderly, or debilitated

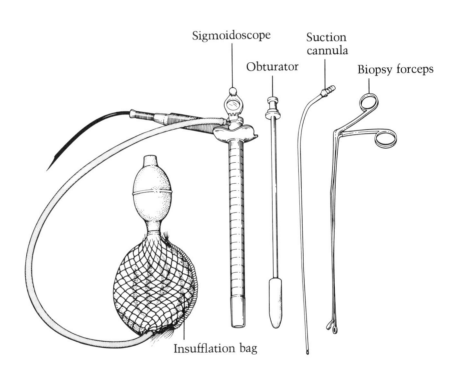

Figure 1
Sigmoidoscopic equipment.

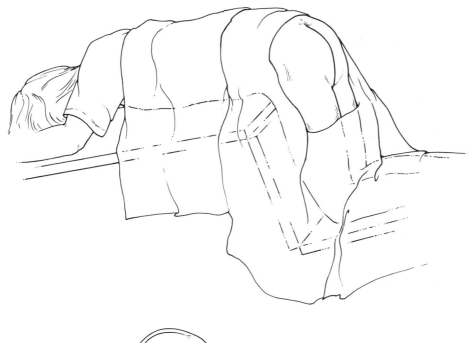

Figure 2
Head-down position.

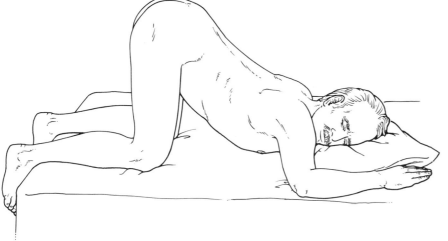

Figure 3
Knee-chest position.

TECHNIQUE

Figures 2, 3, 4

1. **Explain procedure**

2. **Position and drape patient**

3. **Use gloves**

4. **Examine anus and perineum**

5. **Perform rectal exam**

    Use adequate lubrication.

    Exclude stricture or gross anorectal disease.

    Determine direction of anal canal.

Figure 5A, B

6. **Insert sigmoidoscope**

    Place obturator in sigmoidoscope.

    Lubricate distal end of sigmoidoscope and obturator.

    Separate buttocks.

    Gently insert sigmoidoscope into anus about 6–8 cm, aiming for umbilicus.

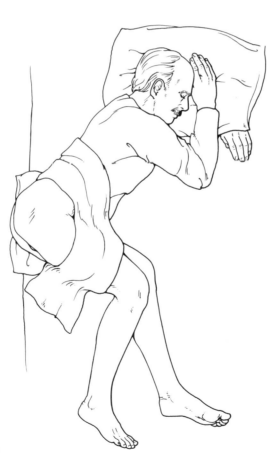

Figure 4
Left lateral Sims's position.

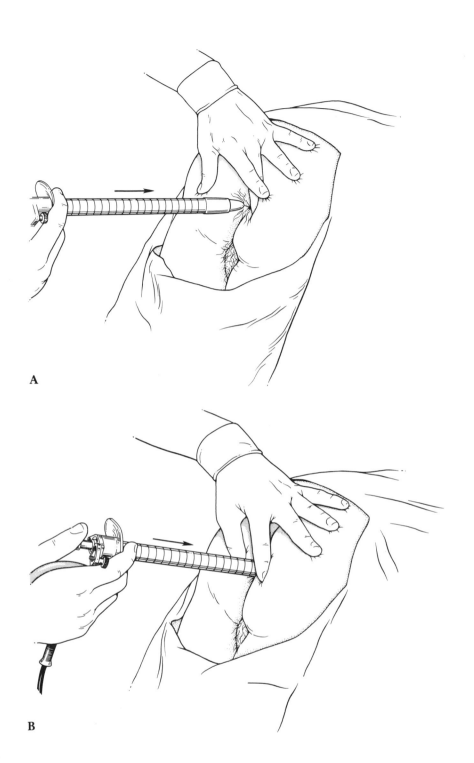

A

B

Figure 5
Insert sigmoidoscope.

Figure 6

7. Advance sigmoidoscope under direct vision

Remove obturator; attach eyepiece.

Advance toward sacrum under direct vision; *never* advance instrument blindly.

Figure 7

Never advance unless lumen clearly visible ahead.

Insufflate air if necessary to distend bowel and facilitate passage.

Gentle pressure against an area of spasm is permissible only if lumen is visible ahead.

8. Examine bowel

Begin examination after sigmoidoscope is advanced as far as is comfortable for patient; do not force beyond this level.

Gentle angulation is permissible to negotiate the rectosigmoid flexure.

Figure 8

Examine bowel as sigmoidoscope is withdrawn.

Use one hand at anus as a fulcrum and sweep instrument around entire circumference of the rectum to visualize all areas.

Keep bowel lumen distended with air to prevent redundant mucosa from obscuring lesions.

Note appearance of mucous membrane: look for ulcerations, bleeding, polyps, tumors, exudates, mucosal injection, hemorrhoids, fissures, and infection.

Note location of lesions: distance from anus and position on circumference of rectum.

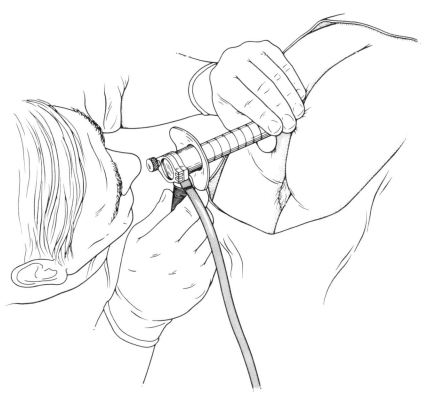

Figure 6
Advance sigmoidoscope
under direct vision.

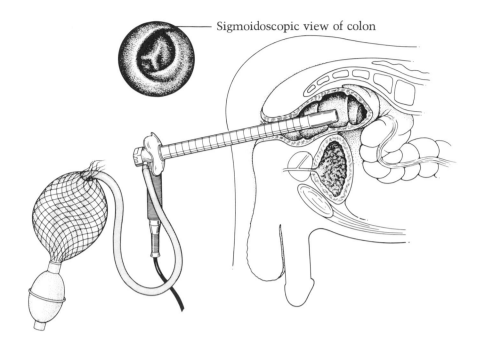

Sigmoidoscopic view of colon

Figure 7
Advance sigmoidoscope
only when lumen clearly
seen ahead (*inset*).

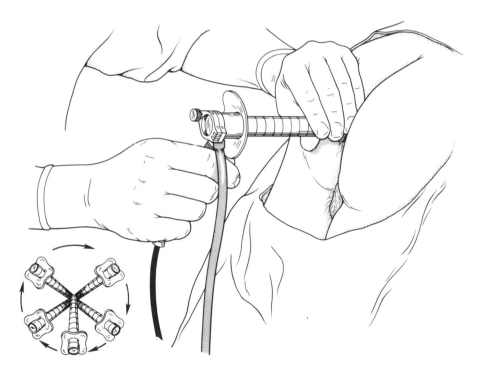

Figure 8
Examine bowel.

257

9. Biopsy suspicious lesions

Remove eyepiece.

Insert biopsy forceps; biopsy lesion.

Avoid full-thickness biopsy of bowel wall.

Cauterize bleeding point with insulated suction tip.

Place specimen in 10% formalin for pathological examination.

COMPLICATIONS

Bowel perforation

Etiology

Excessive force in advancing sigmoidoscope.

Full-thickness biopsy of bowel wall.

Full-thickness necrosis of bowel wall from excessive electrocautery.

Insufflation of excessive air.

Prevention

Do not advance sigmoidoscope unless bowel lumen clearly seen at tip of scope.

Do not use force in negotiating bowel angulation.

Avoid excessive depth of biopsy into wall of bowel.

Do not tear biopsy specimen from bowel; remove only that which comes cleanly away in the forceps.

Biopsy only lesions that are clearly visible.

Use electrocautery for brief periods only.

Insufflate only enough air to produce slight bowel distention; stop when crampy abdominal pain produced.

Excessive bleeding

Etiology

Biopsy of vascular lesion.

Tear of bowel wall.

Intrinsic coagulation defect.

Prevention

Avoid biopsy of obviously vascular lesion.

Carefully cauterize biopsy site that continues to bleed.

Do not force sigmoidoscope.

Do not perform biopsy in presence of coagulation defects.

SELECTED BIBLIOGRAPHY

1. Goligher, J. C. *Surgery of the Anus, Rectum and Colon* (3d ed.). Springfield: Thomas, 1975. Pp. 65–67, 70–85.

   Excellent description of the equipment, techniques, indications for, and complications of proctosigmoidoscopy. Also good descriptions of the technique of digital rectal and anoscopic examination.

2. Spiro, H. M. *Clinical Gastroenterology.* London: Collier-Macmillan, 1970. Pp. 516, 708, 709.

   Short summary of indications for and technique of routine sigmoidoscopy.

28.
Urethral Catheterization

Method of
Timothy B. Hopkins

INDICATIONS

Urinary retention

Monitoring of urine output

Drainage of neurogenic bladder

Obtaining uncontaminated urine specimen

CONTRAINDICATIONS

Acute urethral or prostatic infection

Urethral disruptions due to pelvic trauma

EQUIPMENT (see Appendix for sample kit)

Skin prep

Sterile sponges

Povidone-iodine solution

Sterile field

Towels

Gloves

Catheterization equipment

Water-soluble lubricant

50-ml syringe, catheter tip

Sterile water for injection, 5 ml

Syringe, 5-ml

Sterile saline for injection, 50 ml

#16 or 18 Foley catheter, 5-ml balloon

Closed urinary drainage system

Neomycin 0.5%-fluocinolone 0.025% cream

Adhesive tape, 3-inch

Additional equipment for difficult catheterization

#16 coudé-tip Foley catheter

Lidocaine jelly, 30-ml tube

Curved hemostat

Lidocaine 1%, 20 ml

Zipser clamp

POSITION

Male: supine

Female: supine, "frog leg"

TECHNIQUE—MALE CATHETERIZATION

1. **Retract foreskin**

2. **Prep and drape entire penis**

3. **Use gloves**

4. **Lubricate distal third of catheter**

Figure 1

5. **Insert catheter in urethral meatus**

Gently stretch penis taut to eliminate urethral redundancy.

Figure 2

6. **Advance catheter**

Overcome slight obstruction at sphincter with constant gentle pressure or ask patient to attempt to void.

Advance to balloon sidearm.

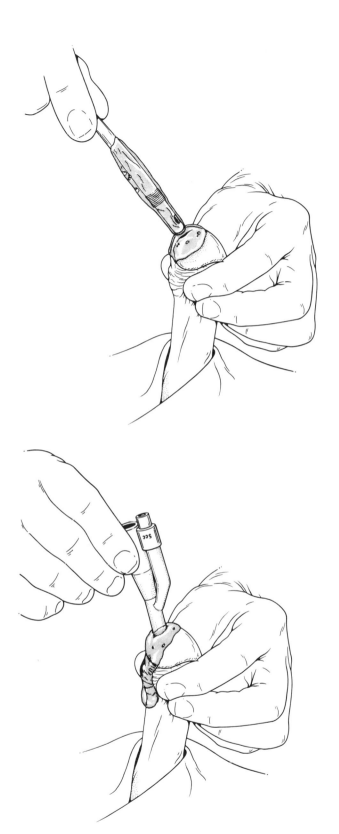

Figure 1
Insert catheter in urethral
meatus.

Figure 2
Advance catheter.

Figure 3

7. Ascertain position of catheter tip

Return of urine through catheter confirms position inside bladder.

If no urine returns, irrigate with 50 ml sterile saline; free fluid return confirms position of catheter in bladder.

8. Inflate catheter balloon

Inject 5 ml sterile water through catheter sidearm.

Figure 4

9. Gently withdraw catheter

Stop when balloon rests against bladder neck.

10. Attach catheter to closed drainage system

Apply small amount of neomycin-fluocinolone cream to catheter-meatal junction.

Tape drainage tubing to medial thigh with 3-inch adhesive tape.

TECHNIQUE—FEMALE CATHETERIZATION

1. Prep and drape labia and urethral orifice

2. Use gloves

3. Expose urethral meatus

Spread labia with thumb and forefinger of left hand.

If meatus is not visualized, place a Kelly clamp in the vagina, open, and retract the vagina posteriorly.

4. Lubricate catheter tip

5. Insert catheter in urethral meatus and advance 4 inches into bladder

6. Ascertain position of catheter tip

Return of urine through catheter confirms position inside bladder.

If no urine returns, irrigate with 50 ml sterile saline; free fluid return confirms position of catheter in bladder.

7. Inflate catheter balloon

Inject 5 ml sterile water through catheter sidearm.

8. Gently withdraw catheter

Stop when balloon rests against bladder neck.

9. Attach catheter to closed drainage system

Apply small amount of neomycin-fluocinolone cream to catheter-meatal junction.

Tape drainage tubing to medial thigh with 3-inch adhesive tape.

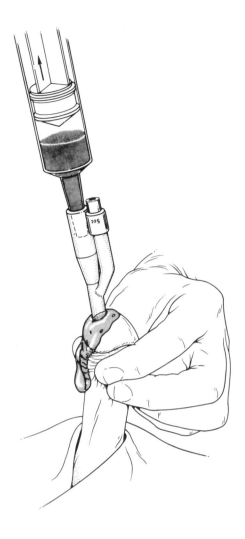

Figure 3
Ascertain position of
catheter tip.

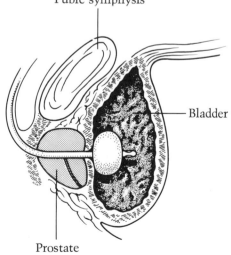

Pubic symphysis

Bladder

Prostate

Figure 4
Gently withdraw catheter.

PROBLEMS IN CATHETERIZATION

Meatal stricture

Dilate stricture with curved hemostat.

Urethral obstruction

Gently instill 20 ml lidocaine 1% with catheter tip syringe.

Place Zipser clamp on penis, wait 5 minutes.

If lidocaine solution instilled easily, fill urethra with lidocaine jelly, using 50-ml catheter tip syringe.

If instillation met with resistance, do not instill lidocaine jelly (possible lubricant embolization).

Repeat attempt at catheterization; use coudé-tip catheter if necessary.

If unsuccessful, proceed with filiforms and followers (see Chapter 29).

Prostatic obstruction

Have assistant direct catheter tip with finger in rectum as catheter is advanced.

Recent prostatic surgery

Use #16 coudé-tip Foley catheter to get over bladder lip.

Direct tip of catheter with finger in rectum.

CATHETER CARE

Wash urethral meatus with soap and water three times daily.

Apply antibiotic-steroid cream to meatus.

Avoid opening drainage system.

COMPLICATIONS

False passage

Etiology

Catheter too small and stiff.

Undue force used in passing catheter.

Urethral stricture.

Prevention

Use appropriate-sized catheter.

Use gentle technique.

Sepsis

Etiology

Catheter balloon inflated in prostatic urethra.

False passage.

Contamination during insertion.

Contamination of closed drainage system.

Preexisting infection.

Prevention

Confirm that catheter is in bladder before inflating balloon.

Avoid catheter tension by taping drainage tubing (not catheter) to medial thigh.

Employ daily catheter care.

Treat urinary tract infections.

Avoid catheterization in presence of known urethral or prostatic infection.

After removal of catheter, treat patient with sulfisoxazole for 7 days.

Urethral stricture

Etiology

Traumatic catheterization.

Urethritis.

Prevention

Use Silastic or Teflon-coated catheters.

Give daily catheter care.

Hematuria

Etiology

Traumatic catheterization.

Preexisting pathology.

Sudden decompression of chronic obstruction.

Prevention

Use atraumatic technique.

Decompress chronic obstruction slowly over several hours.

SELECTED BIBLIOGRAPHY

1. Desautels, R. E.   The causes of catheter induced urinary infection and their prevention. *J. Urol.* 101:757, 1969.

   Analysis of the causes and prevention of catheter-induced urinary tract infections.

2. Foley, F. E. B.   A self retaining bag catheter. *J. Urol.* 38:140, 1937.

   First description of a self-retaining indwelling (urinary bladder) catheter.

3. Kunin, C. M., and McCormack, R. C.   Prevention of catheter-induced urinary-tract infections by sterile closed drainage. *N. Engl. J. Med.* 274:1155, 1966.

   Description of advantages of a closed vs. an open urinary drainage system.

4. Leader, A. J., and Carlton, C. E., Jr.   Urologic Diagnosis and the Urological Examination. In M. F. Campbell and J. H. Harrison (eds.), *Urology* (3d ed.). Philadelphia: Saunders, 1970. Pp. 246–248.

   Exhaustive treatment of all urological techniques.

5. Smith, D. R.   Instrumental Examination of the Urinary Tract. In *General Urology* (7th ed.). Los Altos: Lange, 1972. Pp. 106–111.

   Graphic descriptions of urological techniques.

6. Thomas, G. J.   Urological Instruments. In L. Bransford (ed.), *History of Urology,* American Urological Association. Vol. 2. Baltimore: Williams & Wilkins, 1933. P. 354.

   Reference to first recorded use of hollow tubes of tin and brass as catheters in Egyptian writings of 3000–1440 B.C.

7. Ulm, A. H., and Wagshul, E. C.   Pulmonary embolism following urethrography with an oily contrast medium. *N. Engl. J. Med.* 263:137, 1960.

   Demonstration of potential hazard of instilling lubricants or oily medium into the urethra under pressure in the presence of a urethral stricture.

29.
Passage of Filiforms and Followers

Method of Timothy B. Hopkins

INDICATIONS

Unsuccessful urethral catheterization because of stricture or prostatic hypertrophy

CONTRAINDICATIONS

Acute urethral or prostatic infection

Urethral disruption

EQUIPMENT (see Appendix for sample kit)

Skin prep

  Sterile sponges

  Povidone-iodine solution

Sterile field

  Towels

  Gloves

Catheterization equipment

  Filiforms and followers, graduated sizes

  Closed drainage collection system

  50-ml syringe, catheter tip

  Sterile saline, 50 ml

  Zipser clamp

Topical anesthetic

  Lidocaine jelly, 30-ml tube

  Lidocaine 1%, 20 ml

Figure 1

Dressing

    Adhesive tape, 1-inch, and ½-inch

    Tincture of benzoin

    Neomycin 0.5%-fluocinolone 0.025% cream

POSITION

Supine

TECHNIQUE

1. Prep and drape penis and scrotum

2. Use gloves

3. Instill topical anesthetic

    Gently instill 20 ml of lidocaine 1% into urethra with catheter tip syringe.

    Place Zipser clamp on penis for 5 minutes.

    If lidocaine solution is instilled easily, fill urethra with lidocaine jelly, using 50-ml catheter tip syringe.

    If instillation meets with resistance, do not instill lidocaine jelly (possible lubricant embolization).

Figure 2

4. Pass filiform catheter

    Lubricate all filiforms with lidocaine jelly.

    Pass #4 or #5 olive-tip filiform.

    If obstruction is encountered, rotate and readvance.

    If unsuccessful in entering bladder, leave filiforms at point of obstruction.

    Gently pass one or more curved filiforms alongside the first.

    Advance and rotate each filiform until one passes into bladder.

    Confirm position in bladder by free movement in and out.

    Remove extra filiforms.

5. Pass follower

Figure 3

    Screw #8 or #10 follower onto filiform.

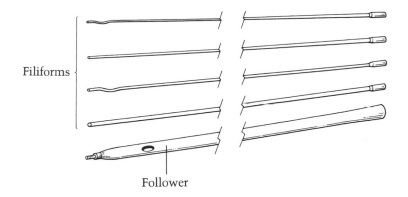

Filiforms

Follower

Figure 1
Filiforms and follower.

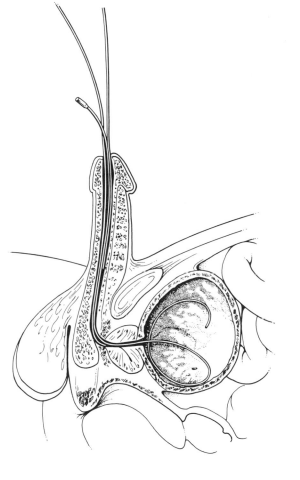

Figure 2
Pass filiform catheters.

Figure 3
Screw follower onto
filiform.

Figure 4

Figure 5

Maintain traction on penis; apply firm steady pressure to advance follower.

If bladder entered (free flow of urine or of irrigation fluid), exchange follower for progressively larger sizes, up to a #20 Fr. or the largest that passes easily.

If impassible obstruction encountered, use smaller follower.

If passage of filiforms and follower unsuccessful, proceed to percutaneous suprapubic cystostomy (see Chapter 30).

6. Secure position of follower, apply dressing

Apply tincture of benzoin to catheter and penis.

Secure with 3 strips of ½-inch tape across junction of catheter and shaft of penis.

Apply 1-inch tape circumferentially (do not constrict penis) around catheter and penis.

Apply neomycin-fluocinolone cream to meatus.

7. Connect to closed drainage system

COMPLICATIONS

False passage

Etiology

Undue force in passing filiform.

Filiform not in bladder when passage of follower attempted.

Prevention

Confirm that filiform is in bladder and not doubled on itself—demonstrate free movement in and out.

Sepsis

Etiology

Acute or chronic urethral infection.

Prevention

Use prophylactic antibiotics before passing filiforms in the presence of urethral infection.

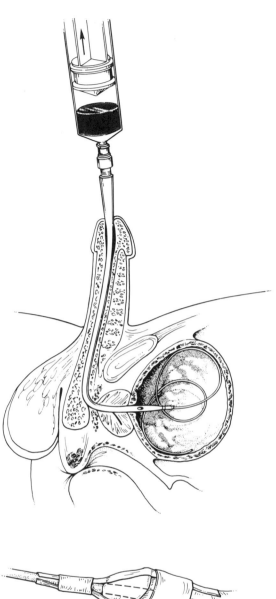

Figure 4
Pass follower, ascertain
position in bladder.

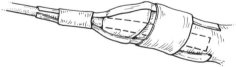

Figure 5
Secure position of fol-
lower, apply dressing.

SELECTED BIBLIOGRAPHY

1. Hand, J. R. Surgery of the Penis and Urethra. In M. F. Campbell and J. H. Harrison (eds.), *Urology* (3d ed.). Philadelphia: Saunders, 1970. Pp. 2594–2596.

   Textbook description of passage of filiforms.

2. Smith, D. R. Instrumental Examination of the Urinary Tract. In *General Urology* (7th ed.). Los Altos: Lange, 1972. Pp. 110–111.

   Brief description and drawing of passage of filiforms.

30.
Percutaneous Suprapubic Cystostomy

Method of Timothy B. Hopkins

INDICATIONS

Acute urinary retention when urethral catheterization and passage of filiforms and followers are unsuccessful

Bladder drainage required in the presence of urethral or prostatic infection

Urethral disruption due to pelvic trauma

CONTRAINDICATIONS

Bladder not palpable

EQUIPMENT (see Appendix for sample kit)

Skin prep

    Prep razor

    Sterile sponges

    Povidone-iodine solution

    Acetone-alcohol solution

Sterile field

    Mask, gloves

    Towels, 4

    Half sheet

Local anesthesia

    Syringe, 3-ml

    Needle, 22-gauge, 1½-inch

    Lidocaine 1%, 5 ml

Cannulation equipment

    Scalpel handle, #3

    Scalpel blade, #11

    Intracath, 12-inch, 14-gauge

    Non-Luer-Lok syringe, 50-ml

    Closed drainage system (sterile IV tubing and empty IV bottle)

    Suture, 2-0 silk on curved cutting needle

    Needle holder

    Suture scissors

Dressing

    Povidone-iodine ointment

    Sterile sponges

    Adhesive tape, 1-inch

POSITION

Supine

Roll under hips

TECHNIQUE

1. Confirm distended bladder by palpation

2. Shave, prep, and drape suprapubic area

3. Use gloves

Figure 1   **4. Infiltrate local anesthetic**

    Midline, 4 cm above pubis

    Down to and including anterior bladder wall

5. Incise skin

    #11 blade, 2-mm stab wound

Figure 2   **6. Insert needle into bladder**

    Place 14-gauge Intracath needle on 50-ml non-Luer-Lok syringe.

    Insert needle through stab wound at 60-degree caudal angle.

    Use short firm thrust to penetrate fascia and enter distended bladder.

    Aspirate urine to ascertain that needle tip is in bladder.

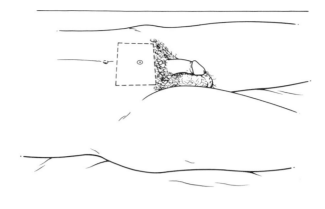

Figure 1
Infiltrate local anesthetic.

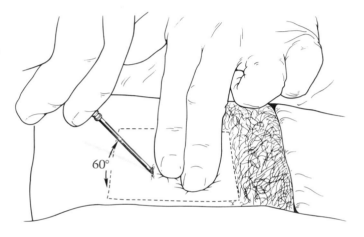

Figure 2
Insert needle into bladder.

7. Cannulate bladder

Remove syringe from needle.

Advance Intracath cannula through needle into bladder.

Withdraw needle from bladder; lock needle and cannula hubs together.

Cover tip of needle with protective device.

Figure 3

8. Recheck cannula position by aspiration

Figure 4

9. Suture catheter in place

10. Attach urinary collection system to catheter

11. Apply sterile dressing

Apply povidone-iodine ointment to skin.

Apply sterile gauze dressing.

Secure catheter and dressing to skin with adhesive tape.

COMPLICATIONS

Hematuria

Etiology

Laceration of submucosal vessel.

Rapid decompression of chronically distended bladder.

Prevention

Gradually decompress chronically distended bladder.

Bleeding usually of little consequence.

Perforation of bowel

Etiology

Bladder not distended.

Improper position of needle.

Prevention

Bladder must be palpable.

Avoid puncture more than 4 cm above pubis.

Avoid puncture off the midline.

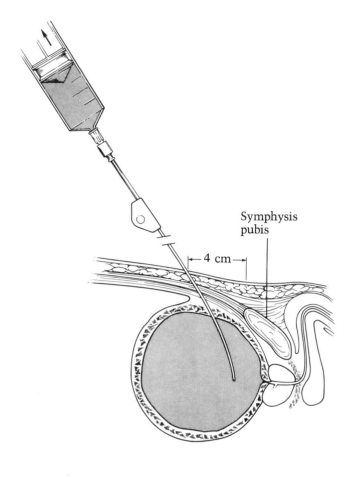

Symphysis
pubis

|← 4 cm →|

Figure 3
Recheck cannula position
by aspiration.

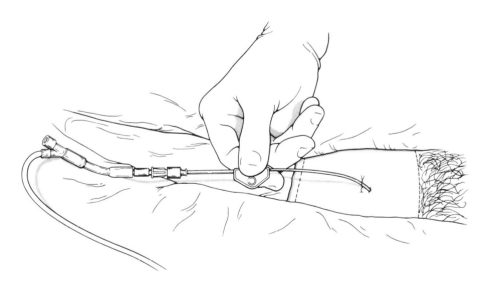

Figure 4
Suture catheter in place.

SELECTED BIBLIOGRAPHY

1. Bonanno, P. J., Landers, D. E., and Rock, D. E. Bladder drainage with the suprapubic catheter needle. *Obstet. Gynecol.* 35:807, 1970.

   Technique and clinical experience in 50 patients with percutaneous suprapubic cystostomy.

2. Campbell, M. F. Surgery of the Bladder. In M. F. Campbell and J. H. Harrison (eds.), *Urology* (3d ed.). Philadelphia: Saunders, 1970. Pp. 2340–2342.

   Technique as described in standard urology textbook.

31.
Peritoneal Dialysis

Method of Peter G. Pletka

INDICATIONS

Renal failure with hyperkalemia, azotemia, or fluid overload

CONTRAINDICATIONS

Ileus

Multiple previous abdominal operations (relative contraindication)

Recent abdominal surgery (relative contraindication)

EQUIPMENT (see Appendix for sample kit)

Skin prep

    Sterile sponges

    Acetone-alcohol solution

    Povidone-iodine solution

Sterile field

    Mask, gown, gloves

    Towels, 4

    or

    Fenestrated drape

Local anesthesia

    Lidocaine 1%, 10 ml

    Syringe, 5-ml

    Needles

        21-gauge × 1½-inch

        25-gauge × ⅝-inch

Dialysis equipment

Peritoneal dialysate (1.5% and 4.25% dextrose in balanced electrolyte solution with heparin, 1000 units/liter)

Peritoneal dialysis catheter with stylette (Stylocath or Trocath)

Dialysis tubing

Scalpel blade, #11

Scissors, suture

Syringe, 10-ml

Injectable saline, 30 ml

Suture, 2-0 silk on curved cutting needle

Needle holder

Dressing

Sterile sponges

Elastoplast

Micropore tape

Denture cup or Dixie cup

Povidone-iodine ointment

Tincture of benzoin

Figure 1

POSITION

Supine

Bladder empty

TECHNIQUE

1. Shave, prep, and drape infraumbilical area

Figure 1

2. Infiltrate local anesthetic

2 inches below umbilicus in midline

Infiltrate from skin to peritoneum

Alternative sites to avoid abdominal scar

Supraumbilical midline

Right or left lower quadrant lateral to rectus sheath

3. Make 4-mm skin incision with #11 blade

Figure 2

Inset

4. Place peritoneal dialysis catheter with stylette in incision

Let stylette protrude ⅛ inch from tip of catheter.

Keep catheter in midline, perpendicular to abdominal wall.

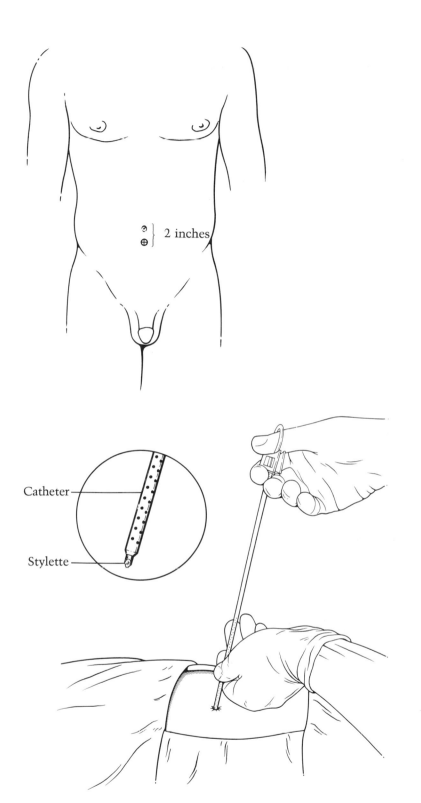

2 inches

Figure 1
Position. Infiltrate local anesthetic.

Catheter

Stylette

Figure 2
Place peritoneal dialysis catheter with stylette in incision.

Figure 3

5. Instruct patient to lift head to tense abdominal wall

6. Insert dialysis catheter into peritoneal cavity

Use both hands, one to provide force, the other to prevent excessive penetration into abdomen.

Slowly advance stylette and catheter until peritoneal cavity entered.

Figure 4A, B

7. Advance peritoneal dialysis catheter

Redirect catheter toward right or left iliac fossa.

Gently advance catheter off stylette, then remove stylette.

Do not advance stylette with catheter.

Ascertain that all catheter perforations are within peritoneal cavity.

If patient experiences pain, withdraw catheter slightly.

8. Confirm intraperitoneal position

Return of free fluid confirms position.

In absence of free fluid, free irrigation of catheter confirms intraperitoneal position.

Figure 5

9. Fix catheter position

Slide fixation clamp to abdominal wall.

Secure catheter with skin suture (optional).

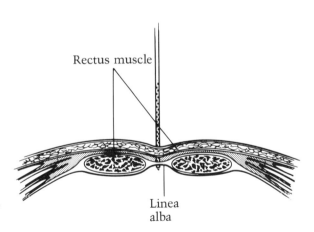

Figure 3
Insert dialysis catheter into peritoneal cavity.

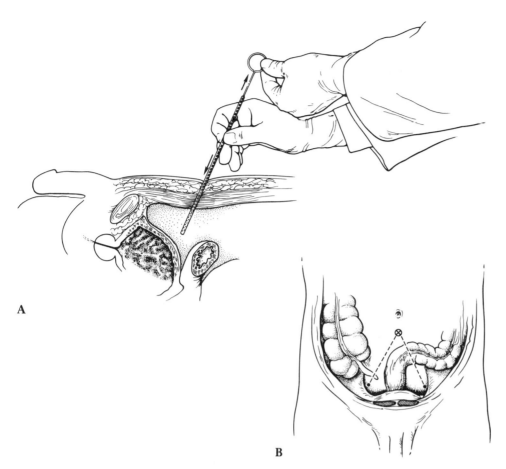

A

B

Figure 4
Advance peritoneal dialysis catheter.

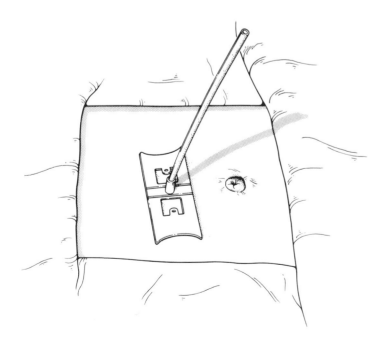

Figure 5
Fix catheter position.

Figure 6   **10. Trim catheter**

Allow 2 inches to protrude from abdominal wall.

Figure 7   **11. Connect catheter to dialysis tubing**

Figure 8   **12. Apply dressing**

Apply sterile gauze dressing around catheter.

Apply Elastoplast to cover dressing.

Place denture cup or Dixie cup to protect catheter.

13. Begin dialysis

Rapidly infuse 2 liters.

If patient experiences discomfort, volume can be reduced to 1 or 1½ liters.

Allow 30-minute dwell time.

Place infusion bottle on floor to permit gravity drainage.

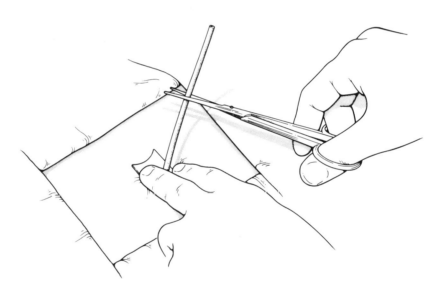

Figure 6
Trim catheter.

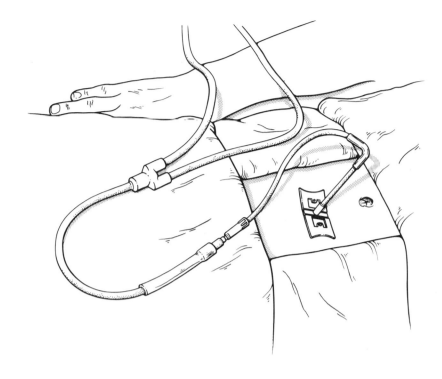

Figure 7
Connect catheter to dialysis tubing.

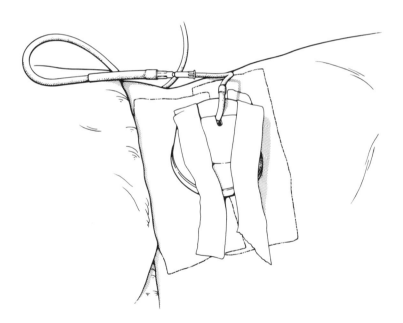

Figure 8
Apply dressing.

COMPLICATIONS

Bleeding from puncture site

Etiology

Laceration of epigastric vessels.

Prevention

Puncture abdominal wall in midline or lateral to rectus sheath.

Bowel perforation

Etiology

Loop of bowel adherent to anterior peritoneum.

Ileus.

Prevention

Do not place catheter through surgical scars.

Do not advance stylette once peritoneal cavity has been entered.

Avoid peritoneal dialysis in presence of dilated bowel.

Intraperitoneal bleeding

Etiology

Laceration of omental or mesenteric vessel.

Prevention

Avoid plunging stylette too deeply; block excessive advancement with lower hand.

Do not advance stylette after peritoneal cavity has been entered.

Perforation of bladder

Etiology

Full bladder.

Puncture site too close to pubis, or angle of insertion too acute.

Prevention

Ascertain that bladder is empty prior to procedure.

Insert cannula perpendicular to abdominal wall.

Perforation of pregnant uterus

Etiology

Advancement of catheter and stylette into uterus enlarged as result of pregnancy.

Prevention

Consider pregnancy a contraindication to midline abdominal paracentesis and lavage.

Respiratory distress

Etiology

Elevation of diaphragm due to abdominal distention.

Prevention

Reduce volume of fluid exchanges.

Abdominal pain

Etiology

Stretching of peritoneum.

Prevention

Add 5 ml lidocaine 1% to alternate 2-liter bottles of dialysate.

Reduce volume of fluid exchanges.

Difficulty infusing dialysate

Etiology

Occlusion of catheter by blood clot or fibrin.

Occlusion of catheter by omentum.

Prevention

Use heparin 1000 units/liter of dialysate.

Place catheter tip in right or left pelvis.

Difficulty draining dialysate

Etiology

Occlusion of catheter by blood clot or fibrin.

Occlusion of catheter by omentum.

Prevention

If catheter is in correct position and not occluded, but not draining adequately, then

Turn patient toward side of catheter, elevate head of bed.

If still not draining, direct catheter to opposite side.

Note: Peritoneal dialysis in patients with multiple previous abdominal operations and associated bowel adhesions is frequently associated with inadequate drainage due to loculation of fluid. Repositioning catheter or reinsertion is sometimes helpful.

SELECTED BIBLIOGRAPHY

1. Boen, S. T. *Peritoneal Dialysis in Clinical Medicine.* Springfield: Thomas, 1964. Pp. 74–90.

   Description of the techniques, indications, and complications of peritoneal dialysis with a review of the literature.

2. Chan, J. C. M., and Campbell, R. A. Peritoneal dialysis in children. A survey of its indications and applications. *Clin. Pediatr.* 12:131, 1973.

   Good review of peritoneal dialysis in children.

3. Ganter, G. Über die Besietigung giftiscuer Stoffe aus dem Blute durch Dialyse. *Muench. Med. Wochenschr.* 70 (II):1478, 1923.

   First description of peritoneal dialysis.

4. Tenckhoff, H. Peritoneal dialysis today: A new look. *Nephron* 12:420, 1974.

   Recent review of peritoneal dialysis.

32.
Percutaneous Femoral Vein Hemodialysis Catheter Insertion

Method of Bruce S. Cutler

INDICATIONS

Hemodialysis for acute renal failure or dialysable toxins

CONTRAINDICATIONS

Iliofemoral thrombophlebitis

Bleeding diathesis

Inguinal sepsis

EQUIPMENT (see Appendix for sample kit)

Skin prep

    Sterile sponges

    Povidone-iodine solution

    Acetone-alcohol solution

Sterile field

    Sterile towels, 5

    Gloves, mask

Local anesthesia

    Syringe, 5-ml

    Needle, 25-gauge $\times$ 1½-inch

    Lidocaine 1%, 20 ml

Cannulation

    Percutaneous femoral hemodialysis catheters, 2

    Guide wire, 0.035-inch (0.88-mm) diameter

    2 syringes, 12-ml

    Dilute heparin saline

      500 units heparin in 100 ml normal saline for injection

    Potts-Cournand needle, 18-gauge thin wall, 2-3/64 inches

    Knife handle, #3

    Knife blade, #11

Dressing

    Sterile sponges

    Povidone-iodine ointment

    Adhesive tape

POSITION

Supine, legs slightly abducted

TECHNIQUE

1. Prep and drape femoral area bilaterally

2. Use gloves and mask

3. Prepare equipment

On sterile field open catheters, guide wire, knife handle and blade.

Fill two 12 ml syringes with heparinized saline.

Figure 1

4. Identify anatomical landmarks

Palpate femoral pulse.

Place first catheter in right femoral vein.

Passage of catheter into inferior vena cava is usually easier from right side.

Figure 2

5. Infiltrate local anesthesia

Inject one fingerbreadth medial to femoral pulse in inguinal crease.

Anesthetize skin and subcutaneous tissue with 5 ml 1% lidocaine.

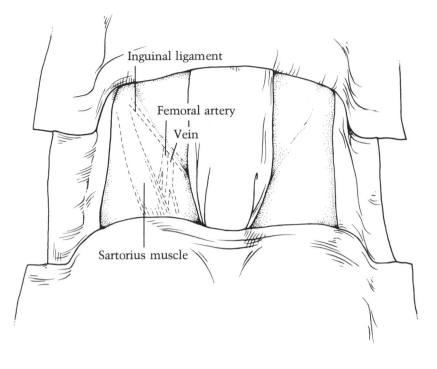

Figure 1
Identify anatomical landmarks.

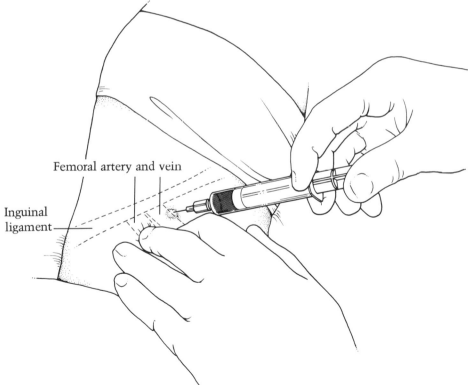

Figure 2
Infiltrate local anesthesia.

Figure 3

Figure 4

Figure 5

Figure 6

6. Puncture vein with Potts-Cournand needle

Engage needle in hub of outer cannula.

Puncture skin one fingerbreadth medial to femoral artery pulsation, in inguinal skin crease.

Angle needle 45 degrees cephalad, parallel with vein.

Do not obstruct hole on end of inner needle.

Slowly advance until blood returns through needle.

Remove inner needle.

Advance cannula 5 mm into vein.

Ascertain blood efflux during 360-degree rotation to ensure entire needle tip is within vein.

Hold forefinger over hub to prevent excessive blood loss.

7. Pass guide wire through cannula

Use soft, flexible end of guide wire.

Gently pass guide wire through cannula into vein.

Caution: Do not advance guide wire if resistance is encountered; laceration of vein may result.

Advance guide wire 20 cm to approximate level of renal veins.

8. Remove cannula

Slide needle out of vein over free end of guide wire.

Do not change position of guide wire.

Caution: Do not pull guide wire back through needle; wire may bend or shear off.

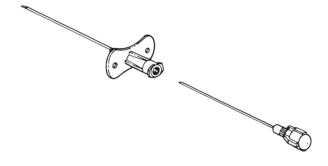

Figure 3
Potts-Cournand needle.

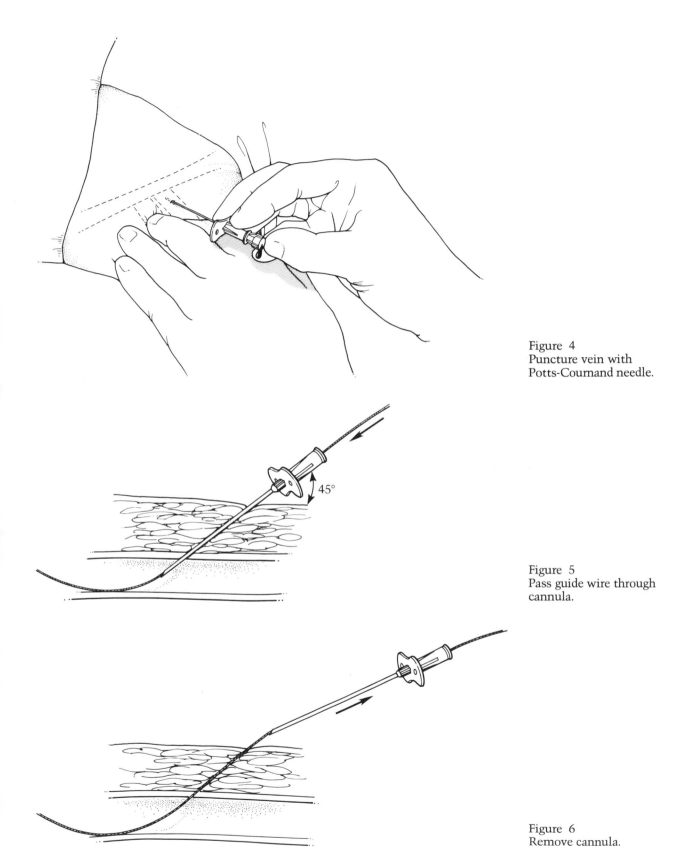

Figure 4
Puncture vein with
Potts-Cournand needle.

45°

Figure 5
Pass guide wire through
cannula.

Figure 6
Remove cannula.

Figure 7

9. Incise skin at puncture site

Make 3-mm skin incision with #11 blade along guide wire at puncture site.

Figure 8

10. Advance hemodialysis catheter over guide wire

Sufficient wire must be left externally so that it will protrude from hub end of dialysis catheter.

Figure 9

Counter traction on skin facilitates passage of dialysis catheter tip through skin and subcutaneous tissue.

Caution: Slide catheter over guide wire; do not allow guide wire to advance with catheter.

Advance catheter so tip lies at level of renal veins (approximately 25 cm) and flexible portion of hub end of catheter remains above skin level.

11. Remove guide wire

Figure 10

12. Flush catheter

Aspirate first, then flush catheter with 10 ml of heparinized saline.

Leave syringe attached until ready for dialysis.

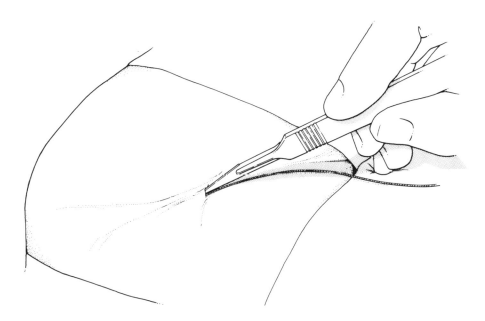

Figure 7
Incise skin at puncture site.

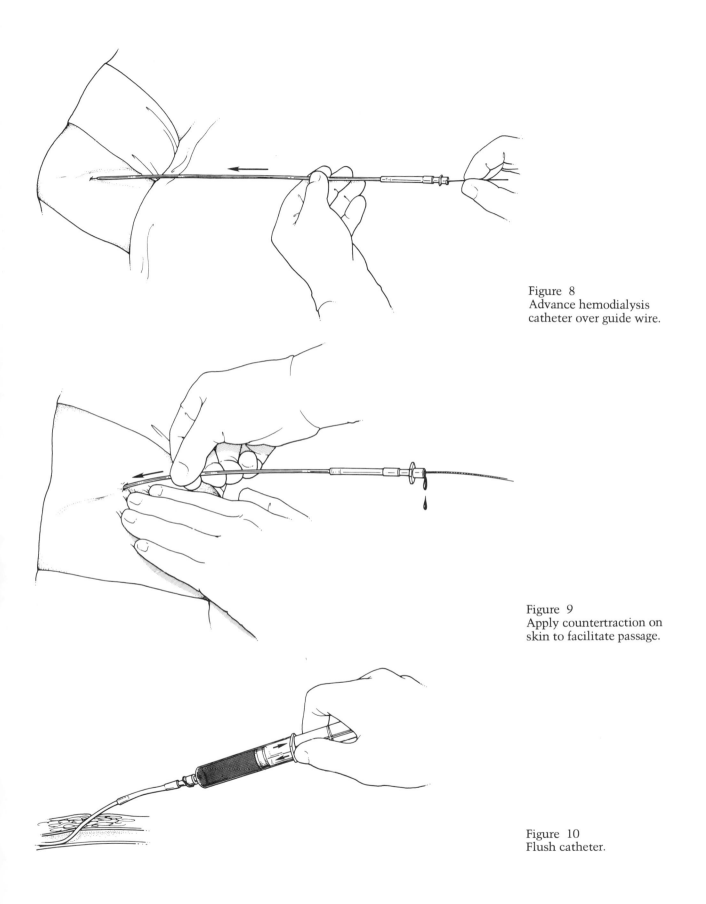

Figure 8
Advance hemodialysis
catheter over guide wire.

Figure 9
Apply countertraction on
skin to facilitate passage.

Figure 10
Flush catheter.

Figure 11

13. Insert second catheter

If hemodialysis equipment requires second catheter, repeat steps 4–12 for puncture of left femoral vein.

Advance tip only to bifurcation of inferior vena cava (approximately 15–18 cm) to prevent contamination of effluent blood with blood returning from dialysis.

Alternatively, two catheters may be placed in same femoral vein. Second puncture should be 2 cm distal to first to prevent laceration of first catheter.

14. Apply dressing

Apply povidone-iodine ointment to puncture site.

Secure catheter to skin with adhesive tape.

15. Attach patient to dialysis machine

With two-catheter technique, the more distal catheter (left) should be used for withdrawal of blood.

Regional heparinization is recommended.

16. Remove catheters

Hold pressure over puncture site for minimum of 5 minutes or until bleeding stops.

Do not leave catheters in situ for subsequent dialysis.

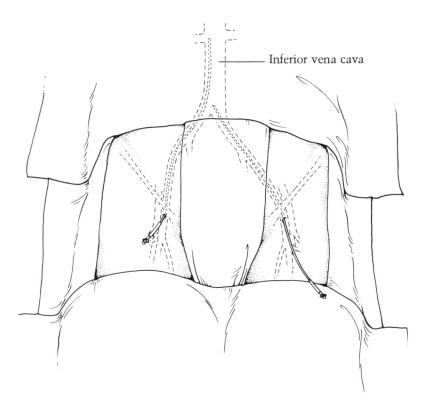

Inferior vena cava

Figure 11
Insertion of second catheter.

COMPLICATIONS

Failure to obtain venous return

Etiology

Thrombosed femoral vein.

Misplaced puncture site.

Management

Withdraw Potts-Cournand needle.

Try again.

Try opposite side.

Puncture of femoral artery

Etiology

Puncture site too far lateral.

Management

Remove needle.

Hold pressure until bleeding stops.

Try again more medially.

High resistance to flow

Etiology

Fibrin deposition on catheter.

Prevention

Fill catheter with heparin saline promptly after placement.

Treatment

Flush forcefully with heparinized saline.

If necessary, pass guide wire through catheter and replace with new catheter.

Retroperitoneal or femoral hematoma

Etiology

   Vein perforation from forceful passage of guide wire or femoral catheter.

   Arterial puncture.

Prevention

   Use only soft end of guide wire.

   Do not advance against resistance.

Iliofemoral thrombosis

Etiology

   Excessive initial trauma.

   Excessive dwell time.

Prevention

   Remove catheters after each dialysis.

SELECTED BIBLIOGRAPHY

1. Nidus, B. D., Matalon, R., Katz, L. A., et al. Hemodialysis using femoral vessel cannulation. *Nephron* 13:416, 1974.

   Experience with 600 acute dialyses. As many as 68 cannulations on a single patient.

2. Serf, B., and Tomasek, R. Hemodialysis by two percutaneous catheters in femoral vein. *Lancet* 1:476, 1964.

   Good description of present venovenous technique.

3. Shaldon, S., Chiandussi, L., and Higgs, B. Hemodialysis by percutaneous catheterization of the femoral artery and vein with regional heparinization. *Lancet* 2:857, 1961.

   First description of original arteriovenous technique.

33.
Diagnostic Paracentesis and Lavage

Method of Wayne E. Silva

INDICATIONS

Diagnosis of intraperitoneal bleeding

Diagnosis of hollow viscus perforation

Treatment of some forms of peritonitis and pancreatitis

CONTRAINDICATIONS

Multiple previous abdominal operations (relative contraindication)

EQUIPMENT (see Appendix for sample kit)

Skin prep

    Sponges, sterile

    Acetone-alcohol solution

    Povidone-iodine solution

Sterile field

    Mask, gown, gloves

    Towels

    Fenestrated sheet

Local anesthetic

    Syringe, 3-ml with 22-gauge needle

    Lidocaine 1%, 5-ml ampule

Paracentesis equipment

    Peritoneal dialysis catheter: Stylocath or Trocath

    Intravenous administration set

    Ringer's lactate, 1 liter

    20-ml syringe

    #15 scalpel blade with handle

Dressing

    Butterfly bandage and Band-Aid

    2.0 silk suture on cutting needle

    Suture scissors

    Povidone-iodine ointment

    Sterile sponges

    Adhesive tape, 1-inch

Figure 1

POSITION

Supine

Bladder empty

TECHNIQUE FOR DIAGNOSTIC PARACENTESIS

1. Shave, prep, and drape infraumbilical area

Figure 1

2. Infiltrate local anesthetic

Infiltrate 2 inches below umbilicus in midline.

Infiltrate from skin to peritoneum.

Do not infiltrate anesthetic into peritoneum (may cause bleeding, giving false positive tap).

Alternative sites to avoid abdominal scar: supraumbilical midline and right or left lower quadrant lateral to rectus sheath

3. Make 4-mm skin incision with #11 blade

Figure 2

Inset

4. Place peritoneal dialysis catheter with stylette in incision

Let stylette protrude ⅛ inch from tip of catheter.

Keep catheter in midline, perpendicular to abdominal wall.

5. Instruct patient to lift head to tense abdominal wall

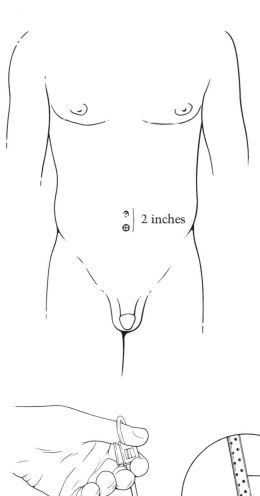

2 inches

Figure 1
Position. Infiltrate local
anesthetic.

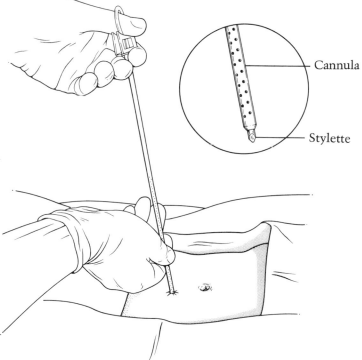

Cannula

Stylette

Figure 2
Place peritoneal dialysis
catheter with stylette in
incision.

Figure 3

6. Insert catheter into peritoneal cavity

Use both hands—one to provide force, the other to prevent excessive penetration into abdomen.

Slowly advance stylette and catheter until peritoneal cavity entered.

7. Advance catheter

Figure 4

Redirect catheter to side most likely to give positive tap.

Gently advance catheter off stylette, then remove stylette.

Do not advance stylette with catheter.

Ascertain that all catheter perforations are in peritoneal cavity.

If pain experienced, withdraw catheter slightly.

8. Slide fixation clamp to abdominal wall

9. Aspirate

Use 20-ml syringe.

Recovery of gross blood or bowel contents constitutes definitive test; remove catheter and apply dressing.

If definitive diagnosis not made, proceed to step 10.

Figure 5

10. Lavage of peritoneal cavity

Connect catheter to intravenous tubing.

Infuse 1 liter Ringer's lactate, clamp IV tubing, and roll patient from side to side to obtain full dispersal of fluid.

Transfer IV tubing to vent hole of IV bottle.

Lower IV bottle to siphon fluid; unclamp tubing.

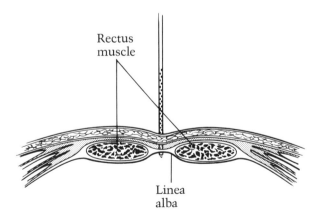

Figure 3
Insert catheter into peritoneal cavity.

Rectus muscle

Linea alba

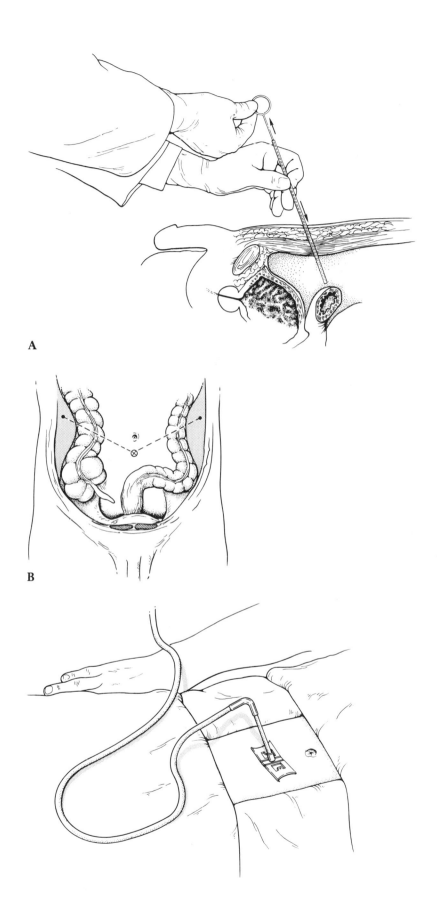

A

B

Figure 4
Advance catheter.

Figure 5
Lavage of peritoneal cavity.

305

11. **Evaluate fluid**

   "Colorimetric test" for evaluation of hemoperitoneum

   Hold IV tubing over newsprint during fluid drainage from abdomen.

   If print cannot be seen: significant injury certain

   If print can be seen but not read: high probability of significant injury

   If fluid bloody but print can be read: equivocal test

   If fluid clear: negative test

   Quantitative tests

   RBC count (done by hemocytometer, not Coulter counter): $> 100,000/mm^3$: high probability of significant injury

   HCT: $> 2\%$—positive test

         1–2%—equivocal test

         $< 1\%$—negative test

   WBC: > 500/cubic ml lavage fluid—positive test

   Amylase: > 200 karoway units/100 ml—positive test
         (normal serum level: 40–160 units/100 ml)

TECHNIQUE FOR THERAPEUTIC LAVAGE

1–7. Same as in preceding technique

8. Secure catheter

   Suture to skin.

   Apply povidone-iodine ointment to puncture site.

   Apply sterile dressing.

9. Begin lavage

   Connect catheter to IV tubing.

   Infuse appropriate therapeutic fluid, allow to drain and repeat.

COMPLICATIONS

Pneumoperitoneum

Etiology

Introduction of air through the catheter.

(Pneumoperitoneum produces no complications but adds difficulty to the interpretation of x-rays. Obtain necessary abdominal x-rays prior to paracentesis.)

Bleeding from puncture site

Etiology

Laceration of epigastric vessels.

Prevention

Puncture abdominal wall in midline or lateral to rectus sheath.

Bowel perforation

Etiology

Loop of bowel adherent to anterior peritoneum.

Ileus.

Prevention

Do not place catheter through surgical scars.

Do not advance stylette once peritoneal cavity has been entered.

Avoid peritoneal dialysis in presence of dilated bowel.

Intraperitoneal bleeding

Etiology

Laceration of omental or mesenteric vessel.

Prevention

Avoid plunging stylette too deeply—block excessive advancement with lower hand.

Do not advance stylette after peritoneal cavity entered.

Perforation of bladder

Etiology

Full bladder.

Puncture site too close to pubis, or angle of insertion too acute.

Prevention

Ascertain that bladder is empty prior to procedure.

Insert cannula perpendicular to abdominal wall.

Perforation of pregnant uterus

Etiology

Advancement of catheter and stylette into uterus enlarged as a result of pregnancy.

Prevention

Consider pregnancy a contraindication to midline abdominal paracentesis and lavage.

SELECTED BIBLIOGRAPHY

1. Bivins, B. A., Jona, J. Z., and Belin, R. P. Diagnostic peritoneal lavage in pediatric trauma. *J. Trauma* 16:739, 1976.

   Description of a modified method of peritoneal lavage for pediatric use.

2. Engrav, L. H., Benjamin, C. I., Strate, R. G., et al. Diagnostic peritoneal lavage in blunt abdominal trauma. *J. Trauma* 15:854, 1975.

   Large clinical study of the technique showing the correlation between lavage results and operative findings.

3. Jergens, M. E. Peritoneal lavage. *Am. J. Surg.* 133:365, 1977.

   Good review of the literature, description of the technique, and explanation of methods of interpretation.

4. Olsen, W. R., Redman, H. C., and Hildreth, D. H. Quantitative peritoneal lavage in blunt abdominal trauma. *Arch. Surg.* 104:536, 1972.

   Description of quantification of blood in lavage fluid, relating it to the incidence of significant injury.

5. Root, H. D., Keizer, P. J., and Perry, J. F., Jr. The clinical and experimental aspects of peritoneal response to injury. *Arch. Surg.* 95:531, 1967.

   Description of the lavage technique and a discussion of the peritoneal response to injury.

6. Sachatello, C. R., and Bivins, B. Technic for peritoneal dialysis and diagnostic peritoneal lavage. *Am. J. Surg.* 131:637, 1976.

   Excellent description of technique with precautions for catheter insertion.

7. Saloman, H. Diagnostische Punktion des Bauches. *Berlin Klin. Wochenschr.* 43:45, 1906.

   Early description of abdominal paracentesis.

34.
Culdocentesis

Method of
Thomas F. Halpin

INDICATIONS

Detection of blood, pus, or intraperitoneal fluid in cul-de-sac

EQUIPMENT (see Appendix for sample kit)

Vaginal preparation

Sterile sponges

Povidone-iodine solution

Long dressing forceps

Drapes, sterile

Local anesthetic

Lidocaine 1%, 10 ml

Syringe, 3-ml

Spinal needle, 22-gauge × 3-inch

Procedure

Graves vaginal speculum

Cervical tenaculum

3-ring handle 10-ml syringe

Spinal needle, 18-gauge × 3-inch

Sterile culture tube

Tubes for clot observation

POSITION

Lithotomy

TECHNIQUE

1. **Perform pelvic and rectovaginal examination**

   Note position of uterus.

   Look for fullness of cul-de-sac.

   Note presence of adnexal masses.

2. **Insert Graves speculum**

3. **Prep posterior vagina**

Figure 1

4. **Elevate cervix**

   Grasp posterior lip of cervix with tenaculum.

   Exert slight upward traction.

5. **Infiltrate local anesthetic**

   Use 22-gauge spinal needle on 3-ml syringe.

   Inject in midline, immediately posterior to vaginal reflection on cervix.

Figures 2, 3

6. **Insert culdocentesis needle**

   Maintain cervical traction with tenaculum.

   Use 18-gauge spinal needle on 10-ml 3-ring syringe.

   Thrust needle quickly through previously raised anesthetic wheal in axis parallel to that of uterus.

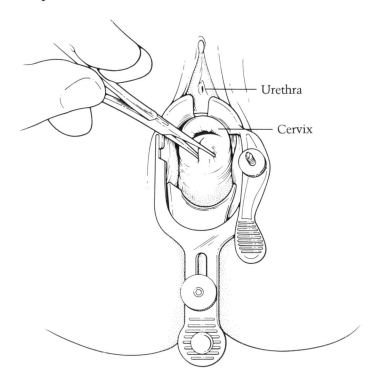

Figure 1
Elevate cervix.

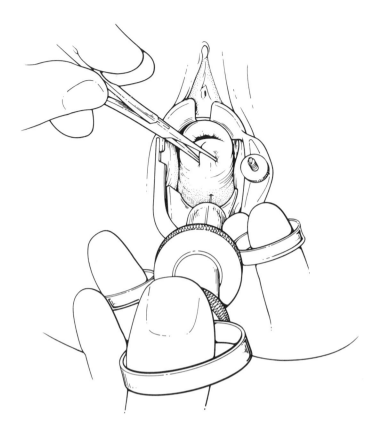

Figure 2
Insert culdocentesis
needle.

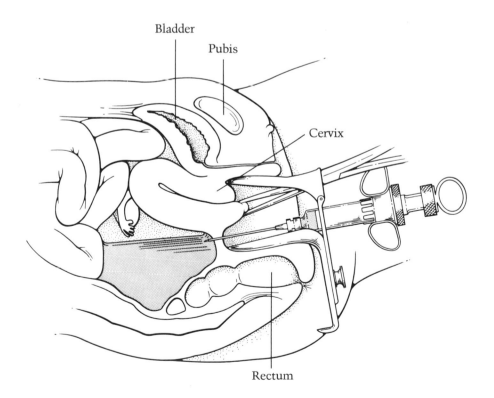

Bladder

Pubis

Cervix

Rectum

Figure 3
Aspirate cul-de-sac.

311

Figure 3

7. Aspirate cul-de-sac

If blood is aspirated, inject it into stoppered glass tube.

Absence of clotting confirms presence of intraperitoneal blood.

If pus is obtained, inject it into sterile culture tube and obtain gram stain.

Culture fluid for aerobic and anaerobic bacteria and for *Neisseria*.

If serous fluid is aspirated, tap is successful, but result of culdocentesis is negative.

If no fluid is obtained, remove needle and repeat step 6.

8. Remove needle

COMPLICATIONS

Aspiration of air or feces

Etiology

Needle directed posteriorly into rectum.

Prevention

Insert needle at apex of cul-de-sac and parallel to axis of uterus.

Intraperitoneal bleeding

Etiology

Needle directed laterally with puncture of mesenteric or pelvic veins.

Prevention

Direct needle in midline.

SELECTED BIBLIOGRAPHY

1. Beacham, D. W., and Beacham, W. D. Culdocentesis. *New Orleans Med. Surg. J.* 103:283, 1951.

   Confirms high diagnostic reliability of culdocentesis in ectopic pregnancy.

2. Decker, A. *Culdoscopy*. Philadelphia: Davis, 1967.

   Technical information on various transvaginal diagnostic and therapeutic procedures.

3. Halpin, T. F. Ectopic pregnancy. *Am. J. Obstet. Gynecol.* 106:227, 1970.

   Review of culdocentesis in diagnosis of ectopic pregnancy.

4. Kelly, H. A. Treatment of ectopic pregnancy by vaginal puncture. *Johns Hopkins Hosp. Bull.* 7:209, 1896.

   First description of evacuation of ruptured ectopic pregnancy through vaginal cul-de-sac—a forerunner of culdocentesis.

5. McGowan, L., Stein, D. B., and Miller, W. Cul-de-sac aspiration for diagnostic cytologic study. *Am. J. Obstet. Gynecol.* 96:413, 1966.

   Large series demonstrating utility of culdocentesis in diagnosis of tumors.

35.
Liver Biopsy

Method of
Gregory L. Eastwood

INDICATIONS

Histological diagnosis of liver disease

CONTRAINDICATIONS

Uncooperative patient

Bleeding disorder

Infection in overlying skin, pleura, right lower lung, or peritoneum

Suspected liver abscess or vascular lesion

Difficulty in determining liver location (as with ascites)

Severe extrahepatic obstruction

EQUIPMENT (see Appendix for sample kit)

Skin prep

Sterile gauze sponges, 10

Acetone-alcohol solution

Povidone-iodine solution

Medicine cup, 30-ml

Rochester-Pean clamp

Sterile field

Sterile towels, 4

Sterile gloves

Local anesthetic

    Syringe, 10-ml

    Needles

        25-gauge × ⅝-inch

        22-gauge × 1½-inch

        20-gauge × 1½-inch

    Lidocaine 1%, 10 ml

Biopsy equipment

    Syringe, 20-ml

    Menghini needle

        1.2-mm for routine biopsies

        1.0-mm for high-risk patients

    Blunted "nail" for proximal portion of Menghini needle

    Stylette (optional)

    Knife blade, #11

    Knife handle, #3

    Injectable saline, 30 ml (should not contain antibacterial preservative if biopsy to be cultured)

    Specimen bottle containing 10% formalin

    Filter paper

Dressing

    Band-Aid

PATIENT PREPARATION

Obtain hematocrit, prothrombin time, partial thromboplastin time, platelet count and bleeding time.

Have patient fast for at least 6 hours before biopsy.

Have patient empty bladder and bowels before biopsy.

POSITION

Figure 1

Supine, right side near edge of bed

Right hand under head; head turned to left

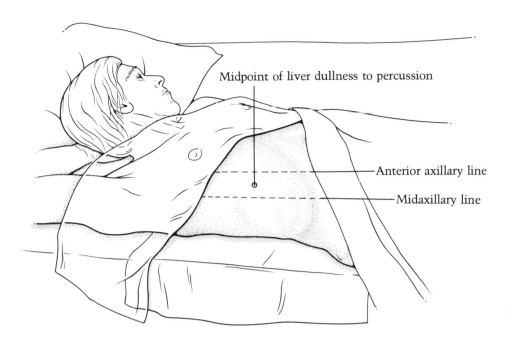

Midpoint of liver dullness to percussion

Anterior axillary line

Midaxillary line

Figure 1
Position, prep, and drape.

TECHNIQUE

1. Identify biopsy site

Intercostal approach: percuss maximal liver dullness between anterior and midaxillary lines after end expiration.

Mark site one intercostal space below.

If liver extends below right costal margin, a subcostal site may be chosen.

If palpable nodule is to be biopsied, mark site directly over nodule.

2. Use sterile gloves

Figure 1

3. Prep and drape 10 cm around biopsy site

4. Have patient practice holding breath for 10 seconds

Full expiration for intercostal approach

Full inspiration for subcostal approach

5. Infiltrate local anesthetic

Figure 2A, B

Anesthetize skin using 25-gauge needle.

Infiltrate to liver capsule with 22-gauge needle.

Do not advance needle through capsule into liver.

Keep needle tract at upper edge of rib.

6. Make 4-mm skin incision with #11 knife blade

7. Assemble biopsy needle and syringe

Figure 3

Fill 20-ml syringe with 10 ml sterile saline.

Insert "nail" into proximal end of biopsy needle to prevent aspiration of biopsy specimen into syringe.

Attach biopsy needle to syringe.

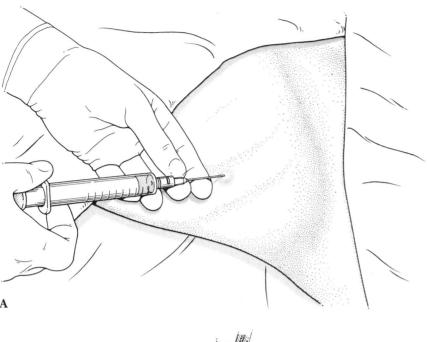

A

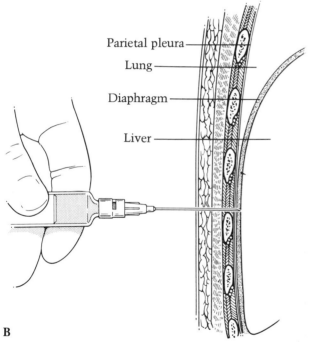

Parietal pleura
Lung
Diaphragm
Liver

B

Figure 2A, B
Infiltrate local anesthetic.

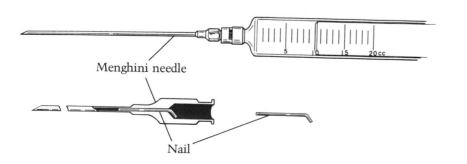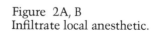

Menghini needle

Nail

Figure 3
Assemble biopsy needle
and syringe.

8. Insert biopsy needle through skin incision

Figure 4

Insert needle parallel to bed toward center of liver (aim toward xiphoid).

Advance needle into but not through intercostal muscles.

Flush needle with 0.2 ml saline.

Figure 4

9. Obtain biopsy specimen

Have patient hold breath at full expiration for intercostal approach, at full inspiration for subcostal approach.

Apply constant suction on syringe.

In a rapid, smooth motion, advance and withdraw needle 4–5 cm. *The total duration of this movement should not exceed 1 second.*

A second biopsy through same incision but at different angle will yield 75% positive results in patients with liver cancer.

10. Fix biopsy specimen

Expel biopsy specimen onto filter paper.

Place specimen into saline or directly into 10% formalin.

11. Apply Band-Aid

POSTBIOPSY CARE

Have patient lie on right side for 2 hours and remain in bed for 8 hours.

Check vital signs frequently.

Obtain hematocrit 4 and 12 hours after biopsy.

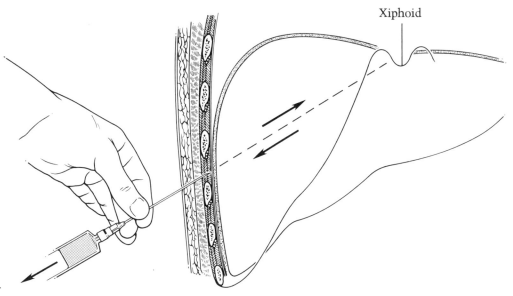

Figure 4
Obtain biopsy specimen.

COMPLICATIONS

Laceration of blood or bile vessels

(Causing hemorrhage, intrahepatic hematoma, hemobilia, bile peritonitis, or hepatoportal AV fistula)

Etiology

Direct trauma to blood and/or bile vessels.

Bleeding disorders.

Bile leaks (most common with obstructive jaundice).

Respiratory motion of liver.

Prevention

Use needle 1.2 mm in diameter or less.

Keep biopsy needle in liver less than 1 second.

Have patient hold breath during biopsy.

Pneumothorax

Etiology

Lung laceration.

Respiratory motion causing laceration if needle passes through lung.

Prevention

Use needle 1.2 mm in diameter or less.

Keep biopsy needle in liver less than 1 second.

Full expiration minimizes chance of needle passage through lung.

Hemothorax

Etiology

Laceration of intercostal artery or vein.

Lung laceration.

Prevention

Pass needle through interspace at upper edge of rib to avoid intercostal vessels.

Injury to other viscera

Etiology

    Improper needle placement.

Prevention

    Precisely determine liver location before biopsy.

Needle fracture

Etiology

    Striking rib with needle.

Prevention

    Before rapid needle thrust, assure intercostal placement.

SELECTED BIBLIOGRAPHY

1. Conn, H. O. Rational use of liver biopsy in the diagnosis of hepatic cancer. *Gastroenterology* 62:142, 1972.

    Liver biopsy is positive in 75% of patients with hepatic cancer.

2. Conn, H. O. Intrahepatic hematoma after liver biopsy. *Gastroenterology* 67:375, 1974.

    Discussion of relationship between needle diameter and development of hematoma.

3. Conn, H. O. Liver biopsy in extrahepatic biliary obstruction and in other "contraindicated" disorders. *Gastroenterology* 68:817, 1975.

    Under certain circumstances, liver biopsy may be performed in the face of some relative contraindications.

4. Edmondson, H. A., and Schiff, L. Needle Biopsy of the Liver. In L. Schiff (ed.), *Diseases of the Liver* (4th ed.). Philadelphia: Lippincott, 1975. Pp. 247–271.

    Review of liver pathology and biopsy methods, including the Vim-Silverman technique.

5. Menghini, G. One-second biopsy of the liver—problems of its clinical application. *N. Engl. J. Med.* 283:582, 1970.

    Standardized technique of liver biopsy emphasizing the importance of small caliber needle.

36.
Soft Tissue
Needle Biopsy

Method of
Wayne E. Silva

INDICATIONS

Obtaining tissue for histological examination, when an incisional biopsy is unnecessary or contraindicated

EQUIPMENT (see Appendix for sample kit)

Skin prep

Sterile sponges

Acetone-alcohol solution

Povidone-iodine solution

Sterile field

Mask, gown, gloves

Fenestrated drape

Local anesthetic

Syringe, 5-ml

Needle, 25-gauge × ⅝-inch

Lidocaine 1%, 5 ml

Figure 1   Biopsy

Vim-Silverman needle

#3 knife handle

#11 scalpel blade

Sterile filter paper

10% formalin

Dressing

Band-Aid

Antibiotic ointment

POSITION

Biopsy site easily accessible

TECHNIQUE

1. Prep and drape biopsy area

Figure 2   **2. Stabilize soft tissue mass with thumb and index finger**

Figure 2   **3. Infiltrate local anesthetic**

Inject skin and proposed biopsy tract.

Figure 3   **4. Incise skin**

Use #11 scalpel blade.

Incise 1–2 mm, at needle insertion site.

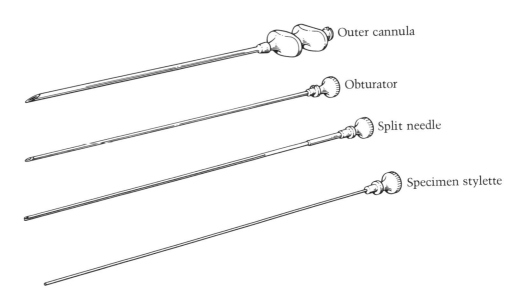

Outer cannula

Obturator

Split needle

Specimen stylette

Figure 1
Vim-Silverman needle.

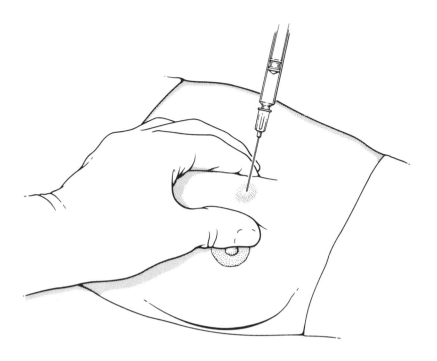

Figure 2
Stabilize soft tissue mass;
infiltrate local anesthetic.

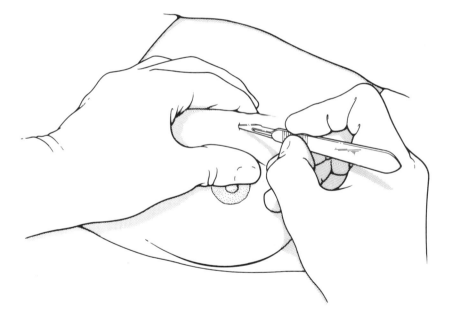

Figure 3
Incise skin.

Figure 4

5. Introduce outer cannula and obturator

Insert to tumor.

Remove obturator.

6. Perform biopsy

Figure 5

Maintain control of mass with thumb and forefinger while inserting split inner needle into tumor (advance until split needle hub is against outer cannula hub).

Figure 6

Advance outer cannula, holding split needle stationary (thereby compressing the two blades of the split needle).

Figure 7

Rotate assembly to break off specimen tip and remove it as a unit.

Figure 8

7. Remove biopsy specimen

Remove split needle from outer cannula.

Separate blades and remove specimen with needle or point of obturator.

Place specimen on sterile filter paper and deposit in 10% formalin.

8. Apply pressure to biopsy site

Hold for 5 minutes to prevent bleeding.

9. Apply dressing

Note: As an alternate method, the Tru-Cut needle (Travenol) may be used conveniently. Excellent instructions are in the package insert.

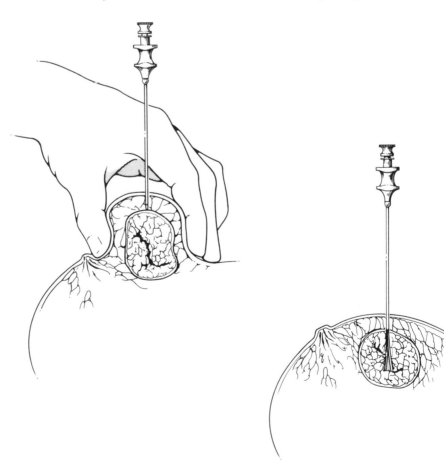

Figure 4
Introduce outer cannula
and obturator.

Figure 5
Perform biopsy: advance
split needle.

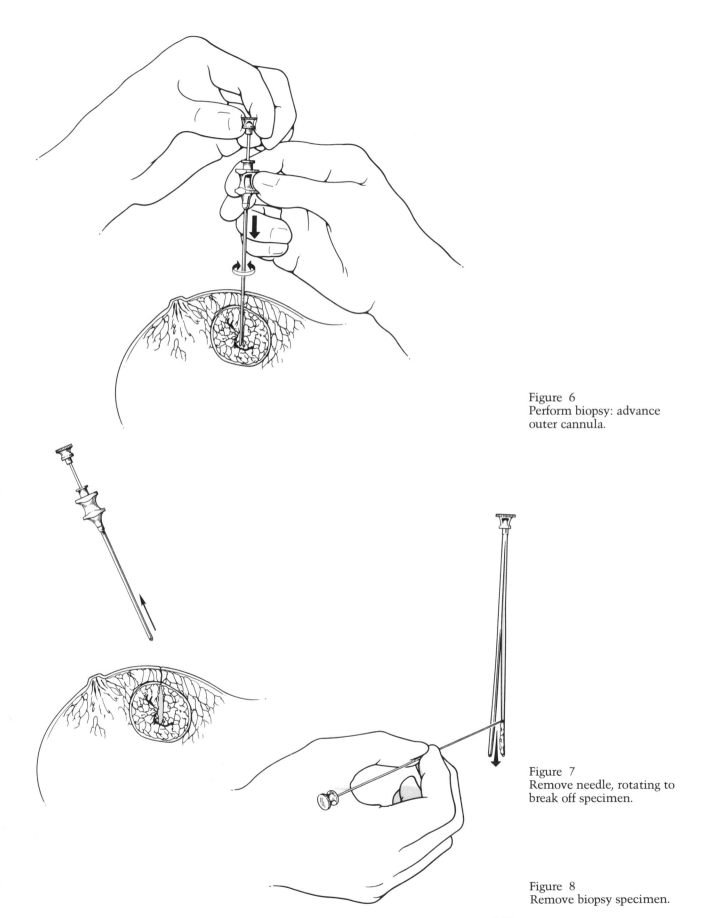

Figure 6
Perform biopsy: advance outer cannula.

Figure 7
Remove needle, rotating to break off specimen.

Figure 8
Remove biopsy specimen.

325

COMPLICATIONS

Dissemination of malignancy

Etiology

The spread of malignant cells is theoretically possible from the mechanical trauma of biopsy.

Prevention

Limit the amount of manipulation and punctures of the tumor.

Excessive bleeding

Etiology

Repeated punctures in a vascular mass.

Clotting defect.

Prevention

Limit the number of biopsies.

Obtain adequate bleeding history, and obtain coagulation studies if indicated.

Apply pressure to biopsy site for 5 minutes.

Infection

Etiology

Inadequate skin preparation or break in sterile technique.

Local infection.

Excessive bleeding in the biopsied tissue.

Prevention

Use proper sterile technique.

Prevent excessive bleeding (see step 2).

Avoid in presence of local infection.

SELECTED BIBLIOGRAPHY

1. Crile, G., and Vickery, A. L. Special uses of the Silverman biopsy needle in office practice and at operation. *Am. J. Surg.* 83:83, 1952.

   Description of uses of the Silverman needle in evaluation of soft tissue, thyroid, and pancreas lesions. Results of 100 consecutive needle biopsies are presented.

2. Deeley, T. J. *Needle Biopsy.* London: Butterworth, 1974.

   Excellent monograph describing the various biopsy techniques and needles available. Good individual chapters on specific biopsy sites, results, and complications.

3. Gault, E. W. The value and limitations of biopsy examination. *Aust. N.Z. J. Surg.* 35:170, 1966.

   Good overview of the subject.

4. Silverman, I. A new biopsy needle. *Am. J. Surg.* 40:671, 1938.

   First description of the Silverman needle.

37.
Bone Marrow Aspiration

Method of
Liberto Pechet

INDICATIONS

Obtaining bone marrow for histological or bacteriological examination

EQUIPMENT (see Appendix for sample kit)

Skin prep

Sterile sponges

Povidone-iodine solution

Alcohol prep sponges

Sterile field

Gloves

Towels

Fenestrated drape

Towel clips

Local anesthetic

Syringe, 3-ml

Needles

25-gauge × ⅝-inch

22-gauge × 1½-inch

Lidocaine 1%, 10 ml

Bone marrow aspiration

Syringe, Luer-Lok, 12-ml

University of Illinois Aspiration Needle (for sternum)

Disposable bone marrow aspiration needle (for iliac crest)

Specimen prep

  Pasteur pipette and bulb

  5–10 microscopic slides, 1-inch × 3-inch

  15–20 coverslips, 1-inch × 1-inch

  10% buffered formalin fixative

  or

  Zenker's solution

Dressing

  Band-Aid

POSITION

Posterior iliac crest aspiration: prone

Anterior iliac crest aspiration: lateral decubitus, hips and knees slightly flexed

Sternal aspiration: supine, no pillow beneath head

TECHNIQUE

1. Prep and drape selected aspiration site

Remove povidone-iodine with alcohol swab.

2. Use gloves

3. Identify anatomical landmarks at selected aspiration site

Figure 1A Posterior iliac crest: center of posterior superior iliac spine

Figure 1B Anterior iliac crest: center of prominence of anterior superior iliac spine, just under lip of crest

Figure 1C Sternum: second intercostal space in midline.

4. Infiltrate local anesthetic

Raise intradermal wheal with 25-gauge needle.

Infiltrate subcutaneous tissue down to periosteum with 22-gauge needle; 2–3 ml lidocaine required.

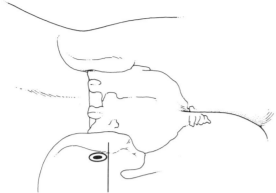

Posterior superior iliac spine

Figure 1A
Posterior iliac crest

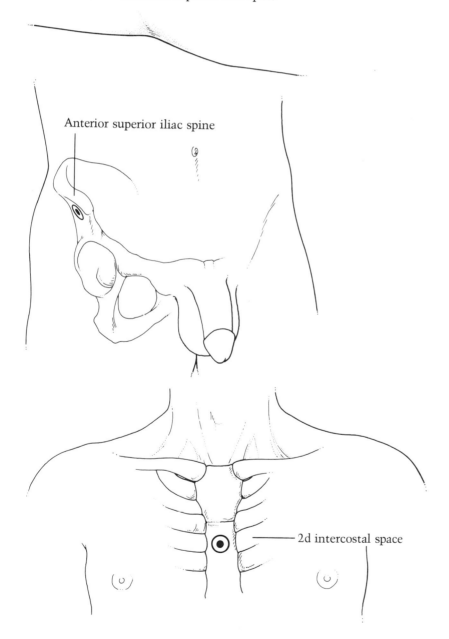

Anterior superior iliac spine

Figure 1B
Anterior iliac crest.

2d intercostal space

Figure 1C
Sternum.

5. Insert bone marrow aspiration needle

Figure 2

Posterior iliac crest aspiration

Use disposable bone marrow aspiration needle.

Hold needle vertically to puncture skin.

Advance needle to center of prominence.

Angle needle 15 degrees caudad.

Forcefully advance into marrow cavity with rotating movements.

Decrease in resistance indicates entry into marrow cavity.

Anterior iliac crest aspiration

Use disposable bone marrow aspiration needle.

Hold needle vertically to puncture skin.

Advance needle to bone.

Angle needle 15 degrees cephalad.

Forcefully advance into marrow cavity with rotating motion.

Decrease in resistance indicates entry into marrow cavity.

Figure 3

Sternal aspiration

Use University of Illinois needle.

Adjust guard to 5–10 mm depth.

Hold needle perpendicular to skin; insert down to bone.

Advance with rotating movement.

Decrease in resistance indicates entry into marrow cavity.

Do not penetrate posterior table of sternum.

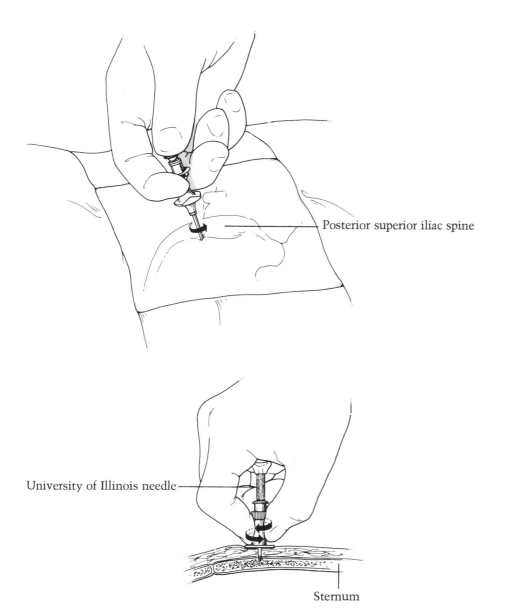

Posterior superior iliac spine

Figure 2
Insert bone marrow aspiration needle: posterior iliac crest.

University of Illinois needle

Sternum

Figure 3
Insert bone marrow aspiration needle: sternum.

6. Aspirate specimen

Attach 12-ml Luer-Lok syringe to needle.

Figure 4A, B

Gently aspirate ½ ml of marrow contents.

Vigorous aspiration is painful and causes dilution of specimen with peripheral blood.

After preparation of smears (see step 7), aspirate a second ½ ml for histological sections.

If inadequate specimen obtained despite correct needle position, proceed to bone marrow biopsy.

7. Prepare specimen

Immediately disconnect syringe and insert stylette into needle.

Arrange several 1-inch × 3-inch glass slides in slanted position.

Figure 5

Allow one drop of aspirate to run down surface of each slide.

Figure 6

Isolate marrow spicules with pipette, and place between coverslips.

Figure 7

Gently crush marrow spicules.

Pull cover slips apart; air dry.

Prepare peripheral blood smear.

Allow second aspirate to clot in syringe, remove plunger, transfer clot to 10% buffered formalin.

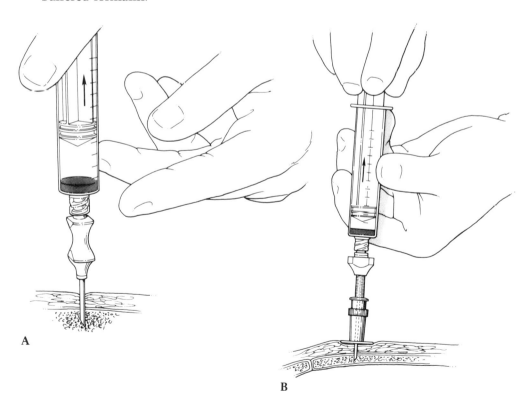

A

B

Figure 4
Aspirate specimen.

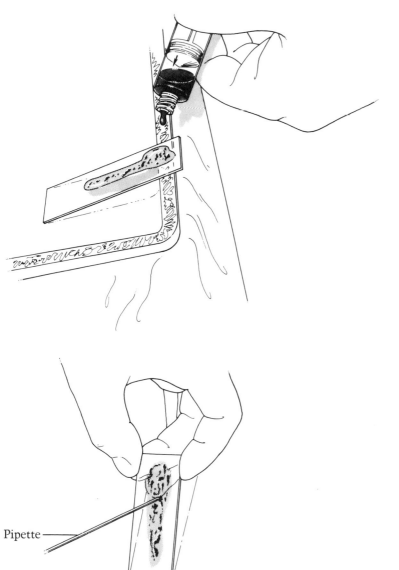

Figure 5
Prepare specimen: place bone marrow on slide.

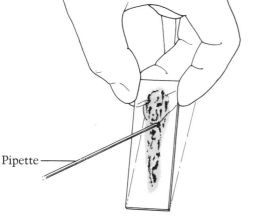

Pipette

Figure 6
Isolate marrow spicules.

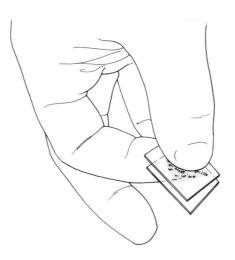

Figure 7
Crush spicules between coverslips.

8. Remove aspiration needle

Apply pressure with sponge until bleeding stops.

Thrombocytopenic patients require longer periods of pressure.

9. Apply Band-Aid dressing

COMPLICATIONS

Bleeding from puncture site

Etiology

Thrombocytopenia, or bleeding diathesis.

Prevention

Local pressure will control most bleeding.

Perform hemostatic evaluation if bleeding diathesis is suspected.

Perforation of aorta

Etiology

Penetration of posterior table of sternum.

Prevention

Use depth guard on University of Illinois needle.

SELECTED BIBLIOGRAPHY

1. Dameshek, W.   Biopsy of the sternal bone marrow. Its value in the study of diseases of blood-forming organs. *Am. J. Med. Sci.* 190:617, 1935.

   First extensive article in English to describe a bedside technique for bone marrow biopsy.

2. Ellman, L.   Bone marrow biopsy in the evaluation of lymphoma, carcinoma and granulomatous disorders. *Am. J. Med.* 60:1, 1976.

   Excellent review of indications for bone marrow biopsies and their findings.

3. Jamshidi, K., and Swaim, W. R.   Bone marrow biopsy with unaltered architecture: A new biopsy device. *J. Lab. Clin. Med.* 77:335, 1971.

   Original description of the Jamshidi needle biopsy, its use and results.

4. Rywlin, A. M.   *Histopathology of the Bone Marrow.* Boston: Little, Brown, 1976.

   Concise book describing techniques of obtaining and staining bone marrow aspirations and biopsies, with good illustrations.

5. Undritz, E.   *Sandoz Atlas of Hematology* (2d ed.). Basel: Sandoz, 1973.

   Excellent illustrations of bone marrow aspirates with description of the technique and useful text on normal and abnormal findings.

38.
Bone Marrow Biopsy

Method of
Liberto Pechet

INDICATIONS

Diagnosis of malignant or granulomatous disease, aplastic anemia, and myeloid metaplasia.

EQUIPMENT (see Appendix for sample kit)

Skin prep

   Sterile sponges

   Povidone-iodine solution

   Alcohol prep sponges

Sterile field

   Gloves

   Towels

   Fenestrated drape

   Towel clips

Local anesthetic

   Syringe, 6-ml

   Needles

      25-gauge × ⅝-inch

      22-gauge × 1½-inch

   Lidocaine 1%, 10 ml

Bone marrow biopsy

   Jamshidi needle (adult or pediatric)

   #3 knife handle

   #11 scalpel blade

Specimen preparation

    10% buffered formalin fixative

    or

    Zenker's solution

Dressing

    Sterile sponge

    Adhesive tape, 1-inch

POSITION

Sternal biopsy not recommended (danger of cardiac injury)

Anterior iliac crest biopsy: lateral decubitus, knees and hips slightly flexed

Posterior iliac crest biopsy: prone

TECHNIQUE

1. **Prep and drape biopsy site**

2. **Use gloves**

3. **Identify anatomical landmarks at selected biopsy site**

    Posterior iliac crest: center of posterior iliac spine

    Anterior iliac crest: just under lip of anterior superior iliac spine

4. **Infiltrate local anesthetic**

    Raise intradermal wheal with 25-gauge needle.

    Infiltrate subcutaneous tissue down to periosteum with 22-gauge needle; 2–3 ml lidocaine required.

5. **Perform bone marrow aspiration first (see Chapter 37)**

Figure 1   6. **Make 3-mm skin incision with #11 scalpel blade**

Figure 2   7. **Prepare biopsy needle**

    Place beveled obturator in needle.

    Engage obturator by locking pin needle with clockwise twist.

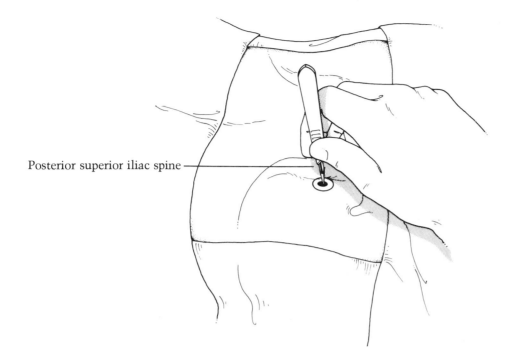

Posterior superior iliac spine —

Figure 1
Make 3-mm skin incision
with #11 scalpel blade.

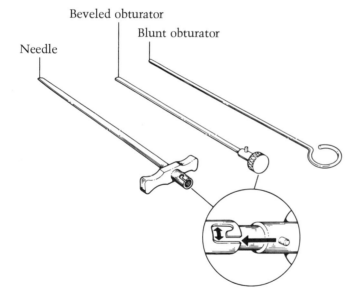

Needle

Beveled obturator

Blunt obturator

Figure 2
Prepare biopsy needle.

Figure 3

8. Insert biopsy needle

Place through incision, perpendicular to bone surface.

Hold needle hub in palm; keep obturator locked.

Advance needle to bone.

Figure 4

9. Obtain biopsy specimen

Posterior iliac crest: angle 15 degrees caudad

Anterior iliac crest: angle 15 degrees cephalad

Advance needle through cortex with forceful rotating movements—decrease in resistance indicates entry into marrow cavity.

Remove obturator.

Advance needle 5 more mm with continued rotation.

Withdraw needle 2–3 mm; do not replace obturator.

Redirect tip at new angle, readvance with rotation, 2–3 mm, to break off biopsy specimen.

10. Remove biopsy needle

Rotate needle during withdrawal.

Apply pressure to biopsy site to control bleeding.

Figure 5

11. Remove specimen from needle

Introduce blunt obturator through distal end of needle.

Push specimen out through hub end of needle onto sterile gauze.

12. Prepare specimen

Make imprints of specimen on coverslips.

Place specimen in 10% buffered formalin or Zenker's solution.

13. Apply dressing

Sterile sponge and 1-inch adhesive tape

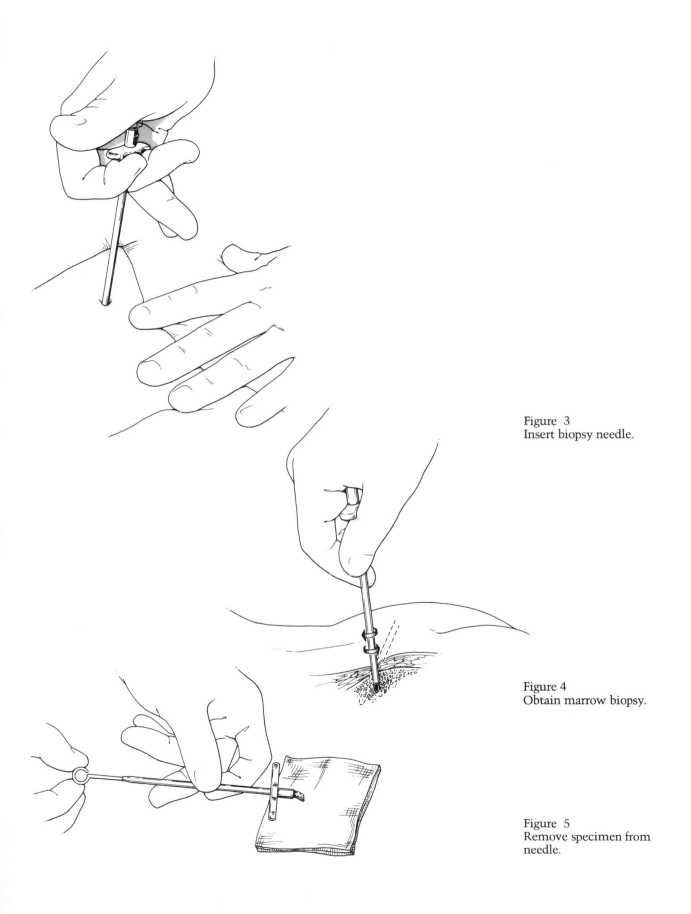

Figure 3
Insert biopsy needle.

Figure 4
Obtain marrow biopsy.

Figure 5
Remove specimen from
needle.

COMPLICATIONS

Bleeding from puncture site

Etiology

Thrombocytopenia or bleeding diathesis.

Prevention

Local pressure will control most bleeding.

Perform hemostatic evaluation if bleeding diathesis is suspected.

SELECTED BIBLIOGRAPHY

1. Dameshek, W. Biopsy of the sternal bone marrow. Its value in the study of diseases of blood forming organs. *Am. J. Med. Sci.* 190:617, 1935.

   First extensive article in English to describe a bedside technique for bone marrow biopsy.

2. Ellman, L. Bone marrow biopsy in the evaluation of lymphoma, carcinoma and granulomatous disorders. *Am. J. Med.* 60:1, 1976.

   Excellent review of indications for bone marrow biopsies and their findings.

3. Jamshidi, K., and Swaim, W. R. Bone marrow biopsy with unaltered architecture: A new biopsy device. *J. Lab. Clin. Med.* 77:335, 1971.

   Original description of the Jamshidi needle biopsy, its use and results.

4. Rywlin, A. M. *Histopathology of the Bone Marrow.* Boston: Little, Brown, 1976.

   Concise book describing techniques of obtaining and staining bone marrow aspirations and biopsies, with good illustrations.

5. Undritz, E. *Sandoz Atlas of Hematology* (2d ed.). Basel: Sandoz, 1973.

   Excellent illustrations of bone marrow aspirates with description of the technique and useful text on normal and abnormal findings.

39.
Lumbar Puncture

Method of Robin I. Davidson

INDICATIONS

Examination of spinal fluid for diagnosis of selected inflammatory, septic, and postinfectious central nervous system disease

Administration of diagnostic and therapeutic agents

CONTRAINDICATIONS

Papilledema or other signs of increased intracranial pressure, or focal neurological signs until mass ruled out

Sepsis in proposed puncture tract (cutaneous infection or osteomyelitis)

Bleeding diathesis or anticoagulant therapy

EQUIPMENT (see Appendix for sample kit)

Skin prep

    Sterile sponges

    Povidone-iodine solution

    Acetone-alcohol solution

Sterile field

    Mask, gloves

    Towels, 2

Local anesthetic

    Needles

        22-gauge $\times$ 1½-inch

        25-gauge $\times$ ⅝-inch

    Syringe, 3-ml

    Lidocaine 1%, 10 ml

Lumbar puncture

Spinal needles (with stylette)

18-gauge × 3-inch

20-gauge × 3-inch

Sterile sponges

3-way stopcock

Manometer

Sterile specimen collection tubes, 3

Dressing

Band-Aid

POSITION

Figure 1   Lateral decubitus with back at edge of bed and knees, hips, back, and neck maximally flexed

Shoulders and pelvis perpendicular to floor

Support under head and, as needed, between iliac crest and inferior costal margin to maintain spine parallel to floor

Alternative position for more accurate localization of midline in patients with obesity, lumbar spondylosis, rheumatoid arthritis, scoliosis, or ankylosing spondylitis.

Figure 2   Sitting on edge of bed, leaning over two bulky pillows on overbed stand

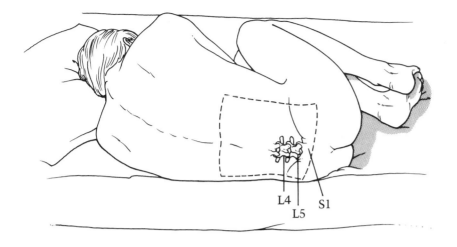

Figure 1
Lateral decubitus position.

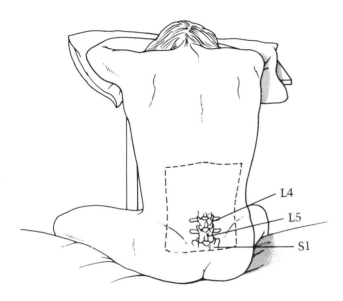

Figure 2
Sitting position.

TECHNIQUE

1. **Use mask and gloves**

2. **Prep and drape at puncture site**

   Midline

   L4–L5 or L5–S1 (iliac crest is at level of L4 spinous process)

3. **Infiltrate local anesthetic**

   Make subcutaneous wheal with 25-gauge needle and infiltrate interspinous area with 22-gauge needle midway between two selected spinous processes.

Figure 3A, B   4. **Insert spinal needle into subcutaneous tissue**

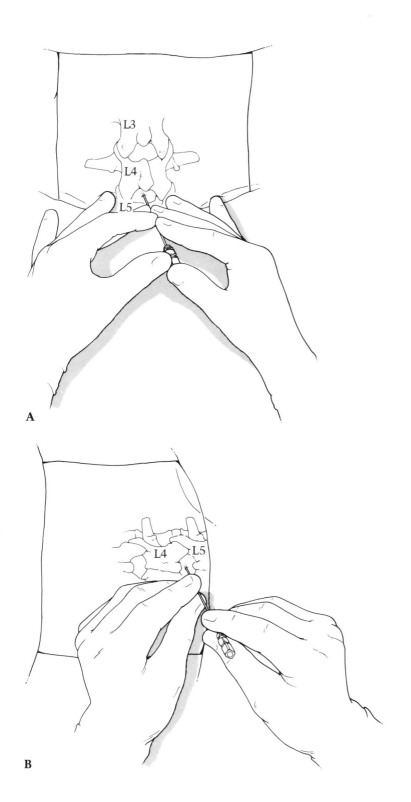

A

B

Figure 3
Insert spinal needle into
subcutaneous tissue.

Figure 4

5. Advance needle into subarachnoid space

Insert 20-gauge needle with bevel parallel to axis of spine.

Use 18-gauge needle in arthritic or obese patient: landmarks are more readily felt with larger needle.

Angle needle 10 degrees cephalad.

Advance slowly until a "give" or "pop" is encountered as needle passes through ligamentum flavum.

At this point (or at a depth of 4 cm in adult if no "give" is felt), remove stylette at each 2-mm interval of needle advancement to check for flow of cerebrospinal fluid.

A second "give" may be felt as needle passes through dura mater.

If bony resistance is encountered, remove needle to subcutaneous layer, change angle, and readvance.

6. If patient in lateral decubitus position, straighten legs and neck

Figure 5

7. Measure opening pressure

Attach manometer and 3-way stopcock.

Use foramen magnum as zero point in sitting position.

Use needle as zero point in lateral decubitus position.

Normal range is 70–180 mm CSF.

Figure 6

8. Collect CSF

Obtain separate samples as indicated for

Cell count and differential.

Protein, sugar, and serological tests.

Gram stain, culture, and sensitivity.

Special studies.

9. Measure closing pressure

10. Remove needle

11. Apply dressing

12. Instruct patient to remain flat in bed for 12–24 hours

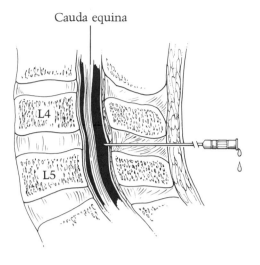

Cauda equina

L4

L5

Figure 4
Advance needle into sub-
arachnoid space.

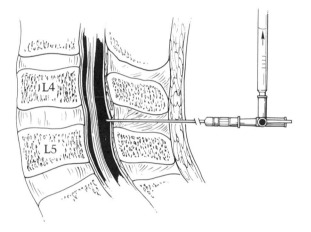

L4

L5

Figure 5
Measure opening pressure.

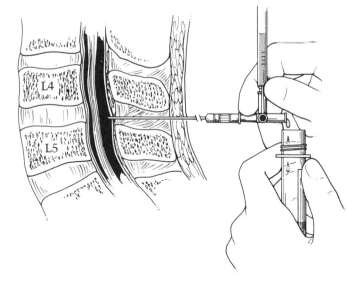

L4

L5

Figure 6
Collect CSF.

347

COMPLICATIONS

Transtentorial or tonsillar herniation

Etiology

Removal of cerebrospinal fluid from below a site of complete or partial impaction of neural tissue, resulting in pressure gradient and progression of herniation.

Prevention

Do not tap in the presence of papilledema or focal neurological signs unless a mass lesion is ruled out.

Exacerbation of paraparesis

Etiology

Removal of CSF caudal to complete intraspinal block.

Prevention

Remove small volume of CSF at time of myelography in patients suspected of intraspinal mass lesion.

Intraspinal epidermoid cyst

Etiology

Introduction of viable epithelial cells into spine canal.

Prevention

Introduce spinal needle with stylette in place.

Meningitis or epidural or subdural empyema

Etiology

Introduction of organisms into subarachnoid space by contaminated needle, inadequate skin preparation, or puncture in the presence of local sepsis.

Prevention

Use meticulous aseptic technique.

Avoid puncture in presence of local sepsis.

Subdural hematoma

Etiology

Removal of large volume of cerebrospinal fluid in an elderly patient, resulting in tearing or avulsion of perforating vein.

Prevention

Remove small volume of fluid slowly in elderly patient.

Prescribe prolonged (24-hour postpuncture) bed rest in elderly patients.

Spinal epidural hematoma or bloody tap

Etiology

Laceration of anterior or lateral epidural venous plexus.

Prevention

Avoid excessively lateral or deep penetration.

Laceration of annulus fibrosus with possible rupture of nucleus pulposus

Etiology

Excessive depth of penetration of spinal needle.

Prevention

Ascertain needle depth by stylette withdrawal at first sign of "give" or at 4-cm depth.

Dry tap

Etiology

Excessively lateral or deep location of needle tip.

Prevention

Accurately determine midline and intraspinal position.

Transient sixth nerve paralysis

Etiology

Removal of large volume of cerebrospinal fluid with traction on the sixth nerve.

Prevention

Remove fluid just sufficient for studies desired.

Transient headache

Etiology

Traction on pain-sensitive basal dura secondary to continued seepage of cerebrospinal fluid.

Occurs in 15–30% of all punctures, most commonly in younger male patient. Lasts 1–10 days, is usually suboccipital in location.

Prevention

Remove volume of fluid just sufficient for studies desired.

Maintain increased hydration postpuncture.

Enforce maintenance of bed rest for 12–24 hours.

Use small-gauge spinal needle: it may reduce cerebrospinal fluid leak.

Transient backache

Etiology

Multiple puncture attempts without local anesthesia with resultant muscle spasm.

Prevention

Adequately infiltrate local anesthetic.

Use single atraumatic pass.

Transient radicular pain

Etiology

Puncture or grazing of nerve root by spinal needle.

Prevention

Insert spinal needle with bevel parallel to axis of spine; if radicular pain encountered, withdraw needle slightly prior to reinsertion.

SELECTED BIBLIOGRAPHY

1. Coben, L. A. Lumbar puncture technique in the adult. *G.P.* 29:110, 1964.

    Contraindications well reviewed.

2. Craigmile, T. K., and Welch, K. Lumbar Puncture and Analysis of Cerebrospinal Fluid. In J. R. Youmans (ed.), *Neurological Surgery* (vol. I). Philadelphia: Saunders, 1973. Pp. 308–325.

    Excellent review, including good discussion of tests on cerebrospinal fluid.

3. DeJong, R. N. *The Neurologic Examination* (3d ed.). New York: Hoeber Med. Div., Harper & Row, 1967.

    Indications, contraindications, technique, and complications with descriptions of Pandy and Queckenstedt tests.

4. Quincke, H. Die Lumbalpunction des Hydrocephalus. *Berl. Klin. Wochenschr.* 28:929, 1891.

    Original article describing measurement of intracranial pressure.

40.
Aspiration and Injection of Joints, Bursae, and Tendons

Method of Carlton M. Akins

INDICATIONS

Diagnosis of joint effusion

Arthrography

Evacuation of hemarthrosis or other effusion

Instillation of drugs

CONTRAINDICATIONS

Skin infection overlying joint

EQUIPMENT (see Appendix for sample kit)

Skin prep

  Sterile sponges

  Acetone-alcohol solution

  Povidone-iodine solution

Sterile field

  Gloves

  Fenestrated drape or half sheet

  Towels

  Towel clips

Local anesthetic

  Syringe, 3-ml

  Needle, 25-gauge × ⅝-inch

  Lidocaine 1%, 10 ml

Aspiration or injection equipment

  Syringes

    5-ml

    10-ml

    30-ml

  Needles

    22-gauge × 2-inch

    20-gauge × 3-inch

    18-gauge × 2-inch

    18-gauge × 3-inch

  Sterile specimen tubes

  Injectable saline

  Drug of choice for instillation

Dressing

  Band-Aid

GENERAL TECHNIQUE

1. Define joint anatomy

Obtain x-rays in two planes.

Correlate x-rays with easily palpable bony landmarks as guides for needle placement.

2. Select approach

Avoid major nerves, vessels, and tendons.

Extensor surfaces are generally preferable.

3. Prep and drape

4. Use gloves

5. Inject local anesthetic along needle tract

6. Perform arthrocentesis

See techniques for specific joints in following section.

Use 18–22-gauge needle of appropriate length.

Avoid injury to articular cartilage with needle.

Send synovial fluid for studies as indicated.

Viscosity

Ropes test (acetic acid clotting)

Cell count

Microscopic examination

Rheumatoid test

LE cells

Culture

Gram stain

Inject medications as indicated.

Remove needle.

7. Apply dressing

Band-Aid

SPECIFIC PROCEDURES

Figure 1   **Glenohumeral (shoulder) joint**

Position

Sitting, arm at side, hand across abdomen

Anterior technique

Insert needle lateral and inferior to coracoid; direct to anterior rim of glenoid.

Figure 2   Posterior technique

Insert needle 2 cm inferior to posterior angle of acromion, direct to posterior rim of glenoid.

Figure 1   **Acromioclavicular joint**

Position

Sitting, arm at side, hand across abdomen

Technique

Palpate joint; insert needle superiorly, direct to lateral end of clavicle.

Figure 1   **Subacromial bursa**

Position

Sitting, arm at side; apply downward traction to flexed elbow.

Technique

Insert needle laterally about 1 cm below tip of acromion.

Direct medially to bursa.

Figure 1   **Bicipital tendon**

Position

Sitting, arm at side

Technique

Insert needle anteriorly at point of maximum tenderness.

Direct needle to bicipital groove.

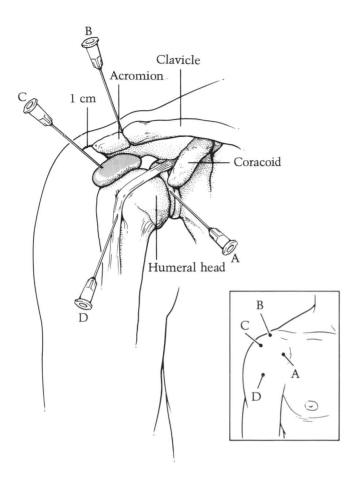

B

Clavicle

Acromion

1 cm

C

Coracoid

Humeral head

A

D

B

C

A

D

Figure 1
A. Glenohumeral (shoulder) joint. **B.** Acromioclavicular joint. **C.** Subacromial bursa. **D.** Bicipital tendon.

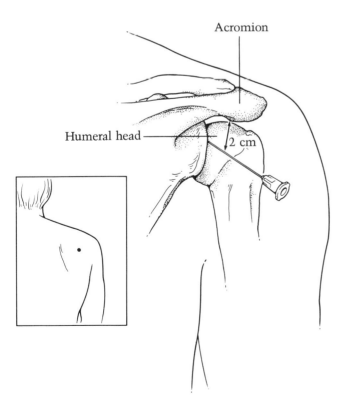

Acromion

Humeral head

2 cm

Figure 2
Glenohumeral (shoulder) joint, posterior approach.

Figure 3

Radiohumeral (elbow) joint

Position

Sitting, flex elbow to 90 degrees; pronate forearm (palm down).

Technique

Insert needle between lateral epicondyle and radial head, direct medially.

Figure 3

Lateral epicondyle

Position

Sitting, flex elbow to 90 degrees; pronate forearm (palm down).

Technique

Insert needle at and direct to point of maximum tenderness.

Figure 3

Olecranon bursa

Position

Flex elbow to 90 degrees.

Technique

Insert needle at posterior tip of olecranon, direct along shaft of ulna.

Figure 4

Radiocarpal (wrist) joint

Position

Flex wrist to 30 degrees; apply traction to hand.

Technique

Insert needle dorsally, distal to dorsal tubercle, medial to extensor pollicis longus tendon, direct volarly to joint.

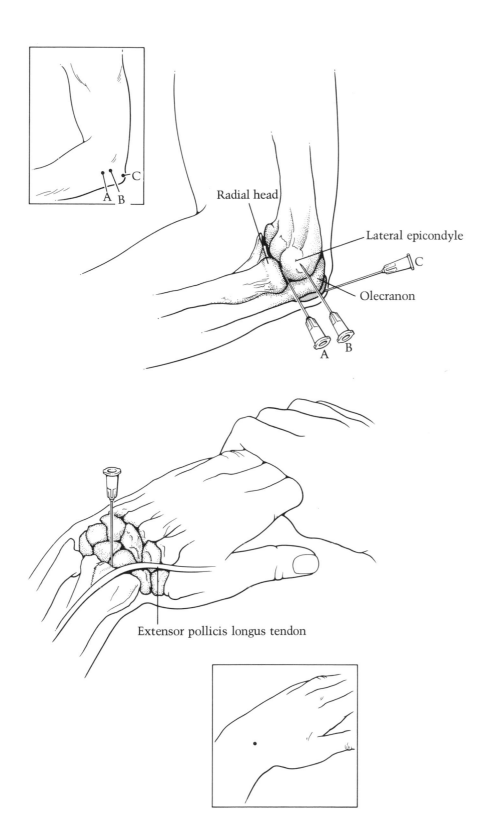

Radial head

Lateral epicondyle

C

Olecranon

A   B

A   B   C

Figure 3
A. Radiohumeral (elbow) joint. **B.** Lateral epicondyle. **C.** Olecranon bursa.

Extensor pollicis longus tendon

Figure 4
Radiocarpal (wrist) joint.

Figure 5

Carpometacarpal (thumb) joint

Position

Oppose thumb to little finger; apply traction to thumb.

Technique

Insert needle proximal to prominence of base of metacarpal, on palmar side of abductor pollicis tendon.

Figure 6

Finger metacarpophalangeal and interphalangeal joints

Position

Flex fingers to 15–20 degrees; apply traction to finger.

Technique

Insert needle dorsally, medial or lateral to extensor tendon.

Hip joint

Figure 7

Lateral approach

Position

Patient supine; hip straight (0 degrees flexion) and internally rotated

Technique

Insert needle anterior to greater trochanter, direct deep to mid portion of Poupart's ligament. Confirm with x-ray.

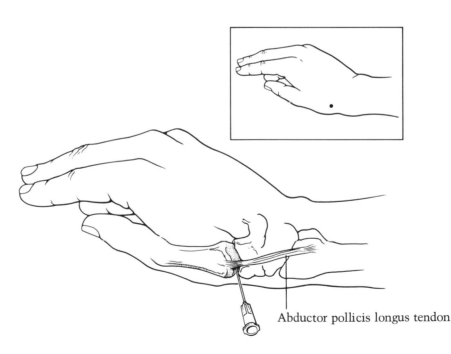

Figure 5
Carpometacarpal (thumb) joint.

Abductor pollicis longus tendon

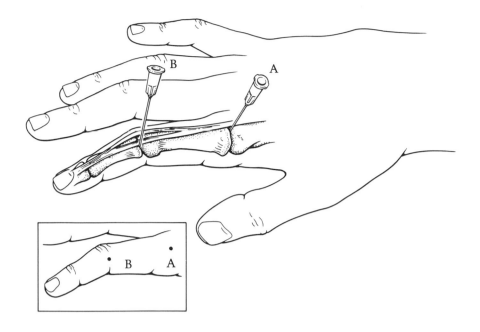

Figure 6
Finger joints. **A.** Metacar-pophalangeal. **B.** Inter-phalangeal.

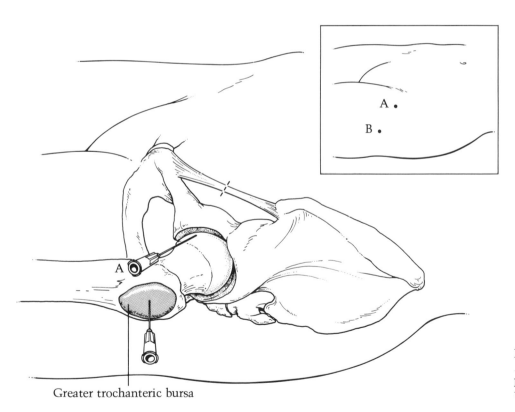

Greater trochanteric bursa

Figure 7
A. Hip joint, lateral ap-proach. **B.** Greater trochan-teric bursa.

Figure 8

Anterior approach

Position

Patient supine; hip straight (0 degrees flexion) and in neutral rotation

Technique

Insert needle at intersection of parasagittal line through anterior superior iliac spine and transverse line through pubic symphysis.

Figure 7

Greater trochanteric bursa

Position

Patient supine; hip straight (0 degrees flexion) and internally rotated

Technique

Insert needle at and direct to point of maximum tenderness.

Knee joint

Figure 9

Anteromedial approach

Position

Supine, knee extended

Technique

Insert needle 1 cm medial to patella; direct to intercondylar notch.

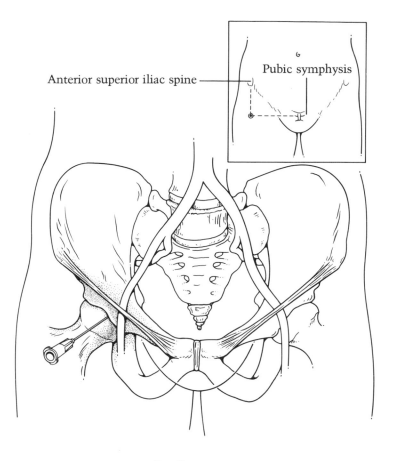

Anterior superior iliac spine ————— Pubic symphysis

Figure 8
Hip joint, anterior approach.

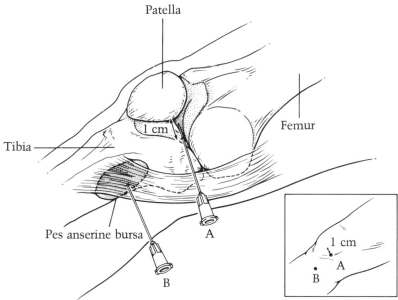

Patella

Tibia

Pes anserine bursa

1 cm

Femur

A

B

1 cm

A

B

Figure 9
A. Knee joint, anteromedial approach. **B.** Pes anserine bursa.

Figure 10   Anterior approach

> Position
>> Flex knee to 90 degrees.
> Technique
>> Insert needle through middle of patellar tendon; direct to intercondylar notch.

Figure 9   **Pes anserine bursa**

> Position
>> Extended knee
> Technique
>> Insert needle at and direct to point of maximum tenderness.

Figure 11   **Tibiotalar (ankle) joint**

> Position
>> Plantar flex foot
> Technique
>> Insert needle medial to anterior tibial tendon, direct to hollow at anterior margin of medial malleolus.

Figure 11   **Metatarsophalangeal and interphalangeal joints**

> Position
>> Flex toes to 15–20 degrees; apply traction.
> Technique
>> Insert needle dorsally, medial or lateral to extensor tendon.

COMPLICATIONS

Hypersensitivity reaction

Etiology
> Allergy to medication.

Prevention
> Exclude allergy by careful history.

Infection

Etiology
> Introduction of bacteria.

Prevention
> Maintain meticulous aseptic technique.
> Avoid passing needle through infected skin.

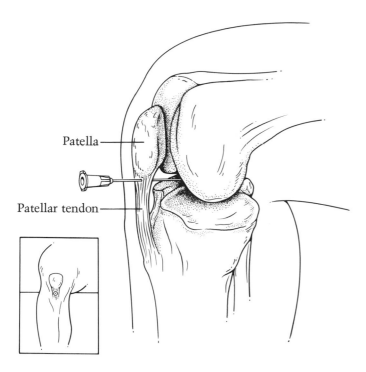

Patella —

Patellar tendon —

Figure 10
Knee joint, anterior approach.

Tibialis anterior tendon

Tibia —

A

Talus —

Extensor hallucis longus tendon —

B

C

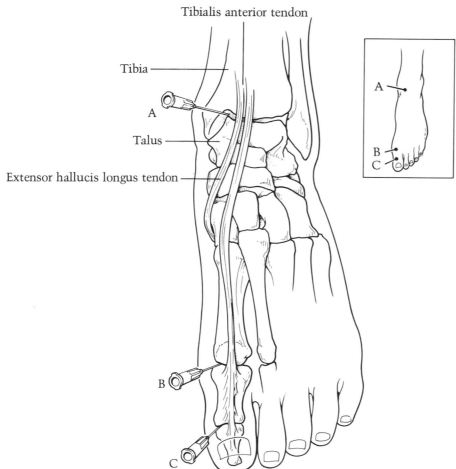

Figure 11
A. Tibiotalar (ankle) joint.
B. Metatarsophalangeal joint. **C.** Interphalangeal joint.

Postinjection flare-up of synovitis (only when corticosteroid injected)

Etiology

Probably due to steroid crystal deposition causing synovitis.

Prevention

Place joint at rest after injection.

Flare-up synovitis may be unavoidable.

Steroid arthropathy

Etiology

Steroid-induced decrease in protein synthesis by articular cartilage.

Prevention

Strictly limit number and dosage of steroid injections.

Minimize frequency and dose of steroid injections (not more than one injection every 3–4 months).

SELECTED BIBLIOGRAPHY

1. Calabro, J. J. Rheumatoid arthritis. *Ciba Clin. Symp.* 23:1, 1971.

   Good overview of rheumatoid arthritis with information on synovial fluid analysis.

2. Hollander, J. L. *Arthritis and Allied Conditions.* Philadelphia: Lea & Febiger, 1972. P. 517.

   The classic Hollander chapter on aspiration and injection.

3. Miller, J. A. Joint paracentesis from an anatomic point of view. Part I: Shoulder, elbow, wrist and hand. *Surgery* 40:993, 1956.

4. Miller, J. A. Joint paracentesis from an anatomic point of view. Part II: Hip, knee, ankle and foot. *Surgery* 41:999, 1957.

   Carefully dissected anatomical specimens with sound recommendations for injection sites.

5. Pruce, A. M., Miller, J. A., and Berger, I. R. Anatomic landmarks in joint paracentesis. *Ciba Clin. Symp.* 16:19, 1964.

   Well-illustrated techniques of specific injection sites.

6. Steinbrocker, O., and Neustadt, D. H. *Aspiration and Injection Therapy in Arthritis and Musculoskeletal Disorders.* Hagerstown: Harper & Row, 1972.

   Good short text on indications and techniques.

7. Sweetnam, R. Corticosteroid arthropathy and tendon rupture. *J. Bone Joint Surg.* 51B:397, 1969.

   Well-reasoned cautions regarding abuse of steroids.

EQUIPMENT

> **Peripheral intravenous cannulation tray**
>
> Intravenous solution, tubing, and stand
>
> Intravenous cannula
>
>> Butterfly needle
>>
>> *or*
>>
>> Plastic cannula
>>
>>> Over-the-needle cannula (Angiocath)
>>>
>>> *or*
>>>
>>> Through-the-needle cannula (Intracath)
>
> Tourniquet
>
> Syringe, 3-ml plastic
>
> Needles
>
>> 25-gauge × ⅝-inch
>>
>> 14-gauge × 1½-inch
>
> Sterile gauze
>
> Alcohol-acetone swab
>
> Povidone-iodine swab
>
> Povidone-iodine ointment
>
> Lidocaine 1%, 5 ml
>
> Adhesive tape, 1-inch
>
> Armboard

EQUIPMENT

Venous cutdown tray

Towels, 4

Towel clips, 4

Syringes

   10-ml

   2-ml

Needles

   22-gauge × 1½-inch

   25-gauge × ⅝-inch

   14-gauge × 1½-inch

Lidocaine 1%, 2 ampules, 5 ml each

Knife handle, #3

Scalpel blades

   #11

   #15

Retractors

   Small self-retaining

   Small rake, 2

Forceps

   Fine-toothed

   Smooth

Scissors

   Suture

   Metzenbaum

   Curved iris

Clamps

   Curved and straight mosquito, 5

Needle holder

Cutdown catheter assortment, Silastic preferred

Ligatures, 3-0 silk

Sutures, skin

Injectable saline, 30-ml vial

ADDITIONAL EQUIPMENT

Gloves, gown, mask

Sterile sponges

Tincture of benzoin

Alcohol-acetone solution

Povidone-iodine ointment

Povidone-iodine solution

Intravenous solution, tubing, and stand

Adhesive tape

EQUIPMENT Chapter 3

Subclavian catheterization tray

2 syringes, 3-ml plastic with 22-gauge × 1½-inch needle

3-ml (non-Luer-Lok) plastic syringe

3-0 silk suture on Keith needle

Lidocaine 1%, 5 ml

Injectable saline, 30 ml

Scissors, suture

Towel clips, 3 disposable

Half sheet

Towels, 3

Sponges, 10

ADDITIONAL EQUIPMENT

Gown, gloves, mask

14-gauge Subclavian Jugular Catheter Set (Deseret)

or

Intracath (Deseret), 12-inch, 14-gauge

Povidone-iodine ointment

Alcohol-acetone solution

Tincture of benzoin

Adhesive tape

    1-inch

    3-inch

Intravenous solution, tubing, and stand

Chapter 4

EQUIPMENT

Subclavian catheterization tray

2 syringes, 3-ml plastic with 22-gauge × 1½-inch needle

3-ml (non-Luer-Lok) plastic syringe

3-0 silk suture on Keith needle

Lidocaine 1%, 5 ml

Injectable saline, 30 ml

Scissors, suture

Disposable towel clips, 3

Half sheet

Towels, 3

Sponges, 10

ADDITIONAL EQUIPMENT

Gown, gloves, mask

14-gauge Subclavian Jugular Catheter Set (Deseret)

or

Intracath (Deseret), 12-inch, 14-gauge

Povidone-iodine ointment

Alcohol-acetone solution

Povidone-iodine solution

Spinal needle, 22-gauge × 3-inch

Adhesive tape

  1-inch

  3-inch

Tincture of benzoin

Intravenous solution, tubing, and stand

Internal jugular vein cutdown tray

Towels, 4

Towel clips, 4

Syringes

  10-ml

  2-ml

Needles

  22-gauge × 1½-inch

  25-gauge × ⅝-inch

  14-gauge × 1½-inch

Lidocaine 1%, 10-ml

Knife handle, #3

Scalpel blades

  #11

  #15

Retractors

  Self-retaining

  Rake, 2

Forceps

  Fine-toothed

  Smooth

Scissors

  Suture

  Metzenbaum

  Curved iris

Clamps

  5, curved and straight mosquito

Needle holder

Cutdown catheter assortment, Silastic preferred, 16-, 18-, 20-gauge

Ligatures, 3-0 silk

Vascular suture, 5-0

Sutures

  Skin

  Subcutaneous

Injectable saline

ADDITIONAL EQUIPMENT

Gown, gloves, mask

Sterile sponges

Petrolatum gauze, 1-inch wide

Alcohol-acetone solution

Povidone-iodine solution

Povidone-iodine ointment

Adhesive tape, 1-inch

Tincture of benzoin

Intravenous solution, tubing, and stand

Chapter 6

EQUIPMENT

Intravenous regional anesthesia tray

Suction source

Oxygen

Means of establishing airway and maintaining ventilation

Blood pressure cuff

Intravenous line in noninvolved arm

Drugs for resuscitation

Lidocaine ½%, 50 ml (*without* epinephrine)

Syringes

   50-ml

   10-ml

Needle, 18-gauge × 1½-inch

Cannula

   Butterfly needle, 21-gauge

   or

   Plastic cannula, 20-gauge (Angiocath or similar over-the-needle cannula)

Injectable saline

Tourniquet

   Double cuff pneumatic tourniquet (single cuff adequate for short procedures)

Rubber bandage (Esmarch or Martin)

Webril or Velband bandage

Sterile sponges

Povidone-iodine solution

Adhesive tape, 1-inch

Inferior vena caval umbrella insertion tray

Sterile sponges

Solution bowl

Towels, 4

Towel clips, 4

Large drapes, 4

or

Laparotomy sheet

Syringe, 5-ml

Needles

    25-gauge × ⅝-inch

    22-gauge × 1½-inch

Knife handle, #3

Scalpel blades

    #10

    #11

Retractors

    Self-retaining (Weitläner)

    Right-angle, 2

Clamps

    5, curved or straight

Scissors

    Suture

    Metzenbaum

    30-degree Potts

Forceps

    Smooth, 2

    Toothed, 2

Vascular tourniquets

    2, 8–10-cm 14 Fr. rubber tubing

    Umbilical tape

    Rummel obturator

Needle holders

    1 vascular

    1 standard

Ligatures

    3-0 silk

    4-0 silk

Sutures

    5-0 vascular

    4-0 silk

    Skin

ADDITIONAL EQUIPMENT

Fluoroscopic table

Mask, gown, gloves

Sterile sponges

Lidocaine 1%, 20 ml

Alcohol-acetone solution

Povidone-iodine solution

Tincture of benzoin

Mobin-Uddin sterile catheter assembly

Adhesive tape, 1-inch

Arterial puncture tray

Glass syringe, 3-ml

Syringe cap

Needles

    20-gauge $\times$ 1½-inch

    23-gauge $\times$ ⅝-inch

Heparin ampule, 1-ml, 1000 units/ml

Sterile sponges

Povidone-iodine solution

Armboard

Nonsterile towel

Adhesive tape, 1-inch

Plastic bag

Crushed ice

Chapter 9 **EQUIPMENT**

Arterial line insertion, percutaneous tray

Syringes

2-ml

10-ml

Needle, 25-gauge × ⅝-inch

Angiocath, 18-gauge, or Medicut cannula, 18-gauge

Stopcock, 3-way

Lidocaine 1%, 1-ml ampule

Heparin, 1 ml of 1000 units/ml

Injectable saline, 30-ml vial

Alcohol-acetone solution

Povidone-iodine solution

Povidone-iodine ointment

Tincture of benzoin

Sterile sponges

Sterile towel

Folded towel, nonsterile

Armboard

Adhesive tape, 1-inch

Arterial pressure transducer

Pressure tubing

Calibrated oscilloscope

Chapter 10 **EQUIPMENT**

Arterial cannula insertion, cutdown tray

Sterile sponges

Towels, 4

Towel clips

Syringes

2-ml plastic

10-ml plastic

Needles

25-gauge. × ⅝-inch

Knife handle, #3

Scalpel blade, #15

Scissors

  Curved iris

  Suture

Forceps, fine-toothed

Clamps, 2 curved mosquito

Retractor, small self-retaining

Needle holder

Lidocaine 1%, 10 ml

Heparin, 1 ml, 1000 units/ml

Injectable saline, 30-ml vial

Ligatures, 3-0 silk

Sutures, skin

ADDITIONAL EQUIPMENT

Armboard

Towel, folded

Adhesive tape, 1-inch

Mask, gown, gloves

Acetone-alcohol solution

Povidone-iodine solution

Povidone-iodine ointment

Tincture of benzoin

Angiocath, 18-gauge, or Medicut cannula, 18-gauge

Stopcock, 3-way

Arterial pressure transducer

Pressure tubing

Calibrated oscilloscope

EQUIPMENT

Balloon flotation catheter kit

Balloon flotation (Swan-Ganz) catheters

　　Double-lumen catheter, #5 Fr. or #7 Fr.

　　or

　　Triple-lumen catheter, #7 Fr. (for CVP and PA pressures)

　　or

　　Quadruple-lumen thermodilution "cardiac output" catheter, #7 Fr.

Strain-gauge pressure transducer, connecting tubing, 3-way stopcocks

ECG monitor (oscilloscope preferred)

Pressure recorder (sensitivity: 1 cm = 5 mm Hg)

Constant infusion system

Portable x-ray or fluoroscope

Cutdown set (see Chapter 2)

or

Subclavian set (see Chapter 3) with Angiocath or other over-the-needle cannula, #16

Introducer: Cook or Desilet-Hoffman introducer of appropriate size for balloon catheter

Scalpel blade, #11

Syringes

　　10-ml

　　5-ml

　　1-ml tuberculin

Needles

　　25-gauge × ⅝-inch

　　21-gauge × 1½-inch

Needle holder

Suture scissors

Towel clips

Towels, 4

Half sheet

Suture, 3-0 silk

Lidocaine 1%, 10 ml

Heparin-saline constant infusion

ADDITIONAL EQUIPMENT

Sterile sponges

Heparinized saline (1000 units/100 ml)

Alcohol-acetone solution

Povidone-iodine solution

Povidone-iodine ointment

Adhesive tape, 1-inch

Intravenous conduit established

Defibrillator

Chapter 12

EQUIPMENT

Temporary transvenous pacemaker placement tray

Pacing catheter, lightweight, semifloating, bipolar. (We prefer Elecath catheter with introducing cannula supplied in kit.)

Suture scissors

Syringe, 5-ml

Needles

 25-gauge × ⅝-inch

 22-gauge × 1½-inch

Skin suture, 3-0

Towel clips

Sterile sponges

Towels, 4

Half sheet

Lidocaine 1%, 10 ml

Alcohol-acetone solution

Povidone-iodine solution

Povidone-iodine ointment

Tincture of benzoin

Mask, gown, gloves

Adhesive tape, 2-inch

ECG machine

Pericardiocentesis tray

Needle-catheter (Subclavian Jugular Catheter Set with metal-hubbed, #14 needle [Deseret])

Stopcock, 3-way

Connecting tubing for stopcock

Syringes

   10-ml

   50-ml

Needles

   25-gauge × ⅝-inch

   21-gauge × 1½-inch

   18-gauge × 2¾-inch spinal

Alligator clip, sterile

Collecting basin, sterile

Culture tubes

Hematocrit tubes

Cytology tubes

Towels

Towel clips

Sterile sponges

Lidocaine 1%, 10 ml

Alcohol-acetone solution

Povidone-iodine solution

Povidone-iodine ointment

Mask, gown, gloves

Adhesive tape, 1-inch

ECG machine, electrically isolated

Chapter 14

EQUIPMENT

Defibrillation and emergency cardioversion tray

Direct current cardioverter with

Oscilloscopic monitor

Selection switches for energy level and storage

Synchronization mode

Electrode paddles (9-cm diameter)

Electrode jelly or saline gauze 4-inch × 4-inch pads

Amnesic drug

Diazepam (Valium), 10 mg/ampule

or

Thiopental sodium (Pentothal), 500 mg/vial

or

Methohexital sodium (Brevital), 500 mg/vial

(Sterile water required to mix with Pentothal and Brevital)

Oxygen with bag-valve-mask device

Venous access

Intravenous cannula (plastic), IV tubing, 5% dextrose

Emergency drugs

Lidocaine 2%

Procainamide, 100 mg/ml

Atropine, 0.4 mg/ml

Isoproterenol, 0.2 mg/ml

EQUIPMENT

Nasotracheal suctioning tray

Suction catheter with finger-occluded suction vent, usually #14 Fr. in adults

Sputum trap

Gloves

Sterile water in container

Specimen container

Water-soluble lubricant

Suction source

Oxygen mask and oxygen source

EQUIPMENT

Chapter 16

Transtracheal aspiration tray

14-gauge (through-the-needle cannula) Intracath

Syringes

   3-ml

   10-ml

Needle, 22-gauge × 1½-inch or 23-gauge × 1-inch

Nonbacteriostatic sterile saline

Lidocaine 1%, 5 ml, *without* epinephrine

Sterile sponges

Fenestrated drape

Alcohol-acetone solution

Povidone-iodine solution

Band-Aid

Gloves

Culture media or transport containers

   Routine

   Anaerobic

Chapter 17

EQUIPMENT

Endotracheal intubation tray

Anesthesia machine or Ambu bag with endotracheal tube/mask connector

Ventilation equipment; depending on needs of patient

Oxygen

Suction with suction catheters and Yankauer suction tip

Venous access

Laryngoscope (curved or straight blade)

Endotracheal tubes (estimated size and one size smaller)

Stylette for endotracheal tube, malleable

Basin with sterile water

Oropharyngeal airway

Clamp, straight mosquito

Scissors

Syringe, 10-ml

Drugs for resuscitation as required

Atropine, 0.4 mg/ml (usually 0.6 mg in adult)

Succinylcholine chloride, 20 mg/ml (usually 1½ mg/kg)

IV solutions

Sterile lubricant, water soluble

Tincture of benzoin

Adhesive tape, 1-inch

Cricothyroid tray

Assortment of standard size tracheostomy tubes (soft cuff)

Basin with sterile water

Delaborde dilator

Suction equipment and tracheal suction catheters

Needle holder

Crile hemostats, 2

Scalpel blade, #11

Knife handle, #3

Syringes, 2 plastic, 10-ml

Needle, 22-gauge × 1½-inch

Towel clips, 4

Sterile sponges

Towels

Fenestrated drape

Mask, gown, gloves

Lidocaine 1%, 10 ml

Acetone-alcohol solution

Povidone-iodine solution

Sutures, 0-silk on curved cutting needle, 2

Catgut ties, 2-0

Chapter 19

EQUIPMENT

Thoracentesis tray

Syringes

    5-ml Luer-Lok, 2

    50-ml plastic Luer-Lok

Needles

    25-gauge × ⅝-inch

    22-gauge × 2-inch

    18-gauge × 2-inch

    15-gauge × 2-inch

Stopcock, 3-way

Rubber tubing attached to stopcock sidearm

Curved clamps, 2

Specimen bowl

Specimen tubes, 3, with stoppers

Lidocaine 1%, 10 ml

Acetone-alcohol solution

Povidone-iodine solution

Fenestrated drape

Sterile sponges

Gloves, mask

Adhesive tape, 1-inch

OPTIONAL

14-gauge Intracath

Syringe, 10-ml non-Luer-Lok

Sterile intravenous tubing

Plasma vacuum bottle

or

Disposable thoracentesis tray with gloves, acetone-alcohol solution, and povidone-iodine solution

Pleural biopsy tray

Cope needle (4 parts)

Syringes

  5-ml

  10-ml

Needles

  25-gauge × ⅝-inch

  22-gauge × 1½-inch

Scalpel blade, #11

Specimen dish with filter paper (sterile)

Lidocaine 1%, 10 ml

10% formalin

Acetone-alcohol solution

Povidone-iodine solution

Sterile sponges

Fenestrated drape

Gloves and mask

Adhesive tape, 1-inch

Chapter 21

EQUIPMENT

Chest tube insertion (closed thoracostomy) tray

Chest tube—type and size depend on purpose and preference

Adults

Pneumothorax

#24 Fr. Argyle straight

Hemothorax or pleural effusion

#32 Fr. Argyle straight or right-angle

Infants

Pneumothorax

#18 Fr. Argyle straight

Hemothorax or pleural effusion

#20 Fr. Argyle straight or right angle

Children

Pneumothorax

Progressively larger size with larger children

Hemothorax or pleural effusion

Largest tube consistent with child's size

3-bottle chest suction

Tubing and connectors (to fit tubing and chest tube)

Syringe, 10-ml

Needles

25-gauge × ⅝-inch

21-gauge × 1½-inch

Needle holder

Suture scissors

Curved clamp (Rochester-Pean)

Knife handle

Scalpel blade, #10

Skin suture, 2-0 silk

Lidocaine 1%, 20 ml

Acetone-alcohol solution

Povidone-iodine solution

Tincture of benzoin

Sterile sponges

Fenestrated drape

Gloves, mask

Petrolatum gauze

Elastoplast, 4-inch

Adhesive tape, 1-inch

Chest tube removal tray

Sterile sponges, 4-inch × 4-inch

Petrolatum gauze

Scissors

Elastoplast, 4-inch

Tincture of benzoin

Chapter 22

EQUIPMENT

Epistaxis tray

Emesis basin

Headlight (or head mirror with light source)

Bayonet forceps

Nasal speculum

Nasal suction (#5 Fraser tip)

Suture scissors

Rochester-Pean clamps, two 7-inch

Gloves

Cautery

   Silver nitrate sticks

   or

   Electric cautery

Cotton pledgets

Selvage gauze, ½-inch or 1-inch

Petrolatum gauze, 3-inch × 36-inch

Surgicel gauze

Umbilical tape

Dental roll

Neosporin ointment

Cocaine, 4%

Catheters, 2 flexible, #12–14 Fr.

Nasogastric tube insertion kit

Nasogastric tube

   For aspiration, Salem sump

   For feeding only, small soft tube or Intracath, 36-inch

Syringe, 50-ml, catheter tip

Emesis basin

Crushed ice in basin

Water-soluble lubricant

Adhesive tape, 1-inch

Glass of water with straw

Sengstaken-Blakemore tube insertion tray

Sengstaken-Blakemore (SB) tube

Nasogastric (NG) tube, #18

Syringe, 50-ml to fit SB tube openings

Clamps, 4 Rochester-Pean

Large scissors

Bulb inflator (from sphygmomanometer)

Manometer (from sphygmomanometer)

Y connector

Connecting tubing

Emesis basin

Glass of water with straw

5-cm cube of foam rubber, cut halfway through

Adhesive tape, 1-inch

Water-soluble lubricant

Chapter 25

EQUIPMENT

Cervical pharyngostomy tray

Right-angle clamp, 7½-inch

Mayo needle holder

Suture scissors

Towel clips

Knife handle, #3

Scalpel blade, #11

Irrigating syringe, 50-ml

Plastic syringe, 3-ml

Needle, 22-gauge × 1½-inch

Nasogastric tube

  #14 for feeding

  #16 or #18 for gastric decompression

Silk suture, 2-0 on curved cutting needle

Towels

Sterile sponges

Fenestrated drape

Gloves

Benzocaine spray, 14% (Cetacaine)

Topical lidocaine, 4%, 5 ml

Injectable lidocaine, 1%, 10 ml

Povidone-iodine solution

Acetone-alcohol solution

Povidone-iodine ointment

Tincture of benzoin

Adhesive tape, 1-inch

Intestinal decompression tray

Intestinal tube (one of the following)

  Cantor

    Single-lumen, gastrointestinal aspiration only

  Kaslow

    Single-lumen, gastrointestinal aspiration only

  Dennis

    Triple-lumen, gastrointestinal sump, and mercury instillation

  Miller-Abbott

    Double-lumen, gastrointestinal aspiration, and mercury instillation

0 silk ligature

Water-soluble lubricant

Metallic mercury, 5 ml

Syringe, 5-ml

Needle, 21-gauge × 1½-inch

Emesis basin

Water in glass with straw

Irrigation syringe, 50-ml

Sigmoidoscopy tray

Sigmoidoscopic table or bed

Patient drape

Lubricant

Gloves

Proctosigmoidoscope, 25–30 cm, with eyepiece, light, obturator, and inflating bulb

Suction tip cannula with tubing

Suction source

Biopsy forceps

Insulated suction tip and electrocautery

Specimen bottle

10% formalin

Chapter 28

EQUIPMENT

Urethral catheterization tray

#16 or 18 Foley catheter, 5-ml balloon

Closed urinary drainage system

Syringes

  50-ml, catheter tip

  5-ml

Towels

Sterile sponges

Gloves

Water-soluble lubricant

Sterile water for injection, 5 ml

Sterile saline for injection, 50 ml

Neomycin 0.5%-fluocinolone 0.025% cream

Povidone-iodine solution

Adhesive tape, 3-inch

ADDITIONAL EQUIPMENT FOR DIFFICULT CATHETERIZATION

Coudé-tip Foley catheter, #16

Curved hemostat

Zipser clamp

Lidocaine jelly, 30-ml tube

Lidocaine 1%, 20 ml

Chapter 29

EQUIPMENT

Filiforms and followers tray

Filiforms and followers, graduated sizes

Closed drainage collection system

50-ml syringe, catheter tip

Sponges, sterile

Towels, sterile

Gloves, sterile

Saline, sterile, 50 ml

Zipser clamp

Lidocaine jelly, 30-ml tube

Lidocaine 1%, 20 ml

Povidone-iodine solution

Tincture of benzoin

Neomycin 0.5%-fluocinolone 0.025% cream

Adhesive tape, 1-inch and ½-inch

EQUIPMENT Chapter 30

Percutaneous suprapubic cystostomy tray

Intracath, 12-inch, 14-gauge

Closed drainage system (sterile IV tubing and empty IV bottle)

Syringes

  3-ml

  50-ml, non-Luer-Lok

Needle, 22-gauge, 1½-inch

Needle holder

Suture scissors

Scalpel handle, #3

Bladc, #11

Prep razor

Suture, 2-0 silk on curved cutting needle

Sterile sponges

Towels, 4

Half sheet

Mask, gloves

Lidocaine 1%, 5 ml

Povidone-iodine solution

Acetone-alcohol solution

Povidone-iodine ointment

Adhesive tape, 1-inch

Chapter 31

EQUIPMENT

Peritoneal dialysis tray

Peritoneal dialysis catheter and stylette (Stylocath or Trocath)

Dialysis tubing

Peritoneal dialysate 1.5% and 4.25% dextrose in balanced electrolyte solution with heparin 1000 units/liter

Syringes

   5-ml

   10-ml

Needles

   21-gauge × 1½-inch

   25-gauge × ⅝-inch

Scissors, suture

Needle holder

Scalpel blade, #11

Sterile sponges, 10

Towels, 4

or

Fenestrated drape

Suture, 2-0 silk on curved cutting needle

1% lidocaine, 10 ml

Injectable saline, 30 ml

Acetone-alcohol solution

Povidone-iodine solution

Povidone-iodine ointment

Tincture of benzoin

Elastoplast

Micropore tape, 1-inch

Denture cup or Dixie cup

Mask, gown, gloves

Percutaneous femoral hemodialysis catheter insertion tray

Percutaneous femoral hemodialysis catheters, 2

Guide wire, 0.035-inch (0.88-mm) diameter

Potts-Cournand needle, 18-gauge thin wall, 2-3/64 inches

Syringes

   5-ml

   12-ml, 2

Needle, 25-gauge × 1½-inch

Knife handle, #3

Knife blade, #11

Sterile sponges

Sterile towels, 5

Gloves, mask

Acetone-alcohol solution

Povidone-iodine solution

Lidocaine 1%, 20 ml

Dilute heparin saline

   500 units heparin in 100 ml normal saline for injection

Povidone-iodine ointment

Adhesive tape

Chapter 33

EQUIPMENT

Midline abdominal paracentesis and lavage tray

Stylocath or Trocath peritoneal dialysis catheter

Syringes

   3-ml with 22-gauge needle

   20-ml

Intravenous administration set

Ringer's lactate, 1 liter

#15 scalpel blade with handle

Suture scissors

Fenestrated sheet

Towels

Sterile sponges

Mask, gown, gloves

Acetone-alcohol solution

Povidone-iodine solution

Povidone-iodine ointment

Lidocaine 1%, 5-ml ampule

2-0 silk suture on cutting needle

Butterfly bandage and Band-Aid

Adhesive tape, 1-inch

Culdocentesis tray

Graves vaginal speculum

Cervical tenaculum

Long dressing forceps

Syringes

   3-ml

   10-ml, 3-ring handle

Spinal needles

   22-gauge × 3-inch

   18-gauge × 3-inch

Sterile sponges

Sterile drapes

Sterile culture tube

Tubes for clot observation

Lidocaine 1%, 10 ml

Povidone-iodine solution

Chapter 35

EQUIPMENT

Liver biopsy tray

Syringes

   10-ml

   20-ml

Needles

   20-gauge × 1½-inch

   22-gauge × 1½-inch

   25-gauge × ⅝-inch

Lidocaine 1%, 10 ml

Sterile gauze sponges, 10

Sterile towels, 4

Medicine cup, 30-ml

Rochester-Pean clamp

Menghini needle

   1.2-mm for routine biopsies

   1.0-mm for high risk patients

Stylette (optional)

Blunted "nail" for proximal portion of Menghini needle

Knife blade, #11

Knife handle, #3

Filter paper

Sterile gloves

Acetone-alcohol solution

Povidone-iodine solution

Injectable saline, 30 ml (should not contain antibacterial preservation if biopsy to be cultured)

Specimen bottle containing 10% formalin

Band-Aid

Soft tissue biopsy tray

Vim-Silverman needle

#11 scalpel blade

#3 knife handle

Syringe, 5-ml

Needle, 25-gauge × ⅝-inch

Sterile sponges

Fenestrated drape

Mask, gown, gloves

Sterile filter paper

Formalin 10%

Band-Aid

Lidocaine 1%, 5 ml

Acetone-alcohol solution

Povidone-iodine solution

Antibiotic ointment

Chapter 37

EQUIPMENT

Bone marrow aspiration tray

University of Illinois Aspiration Needle (for sternum)

Disposable bone marrow aspiration needle (for iliac crest)

Syringes

   3-ml

   Luer-Lok, 12-ml

Needles

   25-gauge × ⅝-inch

   22-gauge × 1½-inch

Towel clips

Pasteur pipette and bulb

5–10 microscopic slides, 1-inch × 3-inch

15–20 coverslips, 1-inch × 1-inch

Sterile sponges

Alcohol prep sponges

Gloves

Fenestrated drape

Towels

Povidone-iodine solution

Lidocaine 1%, 10 ml

10% buffered formalin fixative

or

Zenker's solution

Band-Aid

Bone marrow biopsy tray

Jamshidi needle (adult or pediatric)

#3 knife handle

#11 scalpel blade

Syringe, 6-ml

Needles

   25-gauge × ⅝-inch

   22-gauge × 1½-inch

Towel clips

Sterile sponges

Alcohol prep sponges

Towels

Fenestrated drape

Gloves

Povidone-iodine solution

Lidocaine 1%, 10 ml

10% buffered formalin fixative

or

Zenker's solution

Adhesive tape, 1-inch

Chapter 39

EQUIPMENT

Lumbar puncture tray

3-way stopcock

Manometer

Sterile specimen collection tubes, 3

Needles

    22-gauge × 1½-inch

    25-gauge × ⅝-inch

Spinal needles (with stylette)

    18-gauge × 3-inch

    20-gauge × 3-inch

Syringe, 3-ml

Towels, 2

Sterile sponges

Mask, gloves

Lidocaine 1%, 10 ml

Povidone-iodine solution

Acetone-alcohol solution

Band-Aid

Arthrocentesis tray

Syringes

   3-ml

   5-ml

   10-ml

   30-ml

Needles

   25-gauge × ⅝-inch

   22-gauge × 2-inch

   20-gauge × 3-inch

   18-gauge × 2-inch

   18-gauge × 3-inch

Sterile sponges

Fenestrated drape or half sheet

Towels

Towel clips

Gloves

Acetone-alcohol solution

Povidone-iodine solution

Lidocaine 1%, 10 ml

Injectable saline

Drug of choice for instillation

Sterile specimen tubes

Band-Aid

Index

BELMONT COLLEGE LIBRARY

6666   57